RESPIRATORY THERAPY COMPETENCY EVALUATION MANUAL

RESPIRATORY THERAPY COMPETENCY EVALUATION MANUAL

Craig L. Scanlan, Ed.D., R.R.T.
Associate Professor and Chairman
Department of Health Education, Evaluation and Research
School of Health Related Professions
University of Medicine and Dentistry of New Jersey
Newark, New Jersey

George A. West, M.S., R.R.T.
Vice President and Consultant
Continuing Care Associates
Formerly
Director of Respiratory Care and Associate in Anesthesia
Massachusetts General Hospital and Harvard Medical School
Boston, Massachusetts

Gerald K. Dolan, M.S., R.R.T.
Associate Professor and Director
Respiratory Therapy Program
Ferris State College
Big Rapids, Michigan

Philip A. von der Heydt, M.Ed., R.R.T.
Executive Director
Joint Review Committee for Respiratory Therapy Education
Euless, Texas

Blackwell Scientific Publications, Inc.
Boston   Oxford   London   Edinburgh   Palo Alto   Melbourne

Blackwell Scientific Publications

Editorial offices at:
Osney Mead, Oxford OX2 0EL, England
8 John Street, London WC1N 2ES, England
23 Ainslie Place, Edinburgh EH3 6AJ, Scotland
107 Barry Street, Carlton, Victoria 3053, Australia
667 Lytton Avenue, Palo Alto, CA 94301, USA

Distributors:
USA and Canada
        Blackwell Mosby Book Distributors
        11830 Westline Industrial Drive
        St. Louis, Missouri 63146

Australia
        Blackwell Scientific Book Distributors, Pty., Ltd.
        107 Barry Street
        Carlton, Victoria, 3053, Australia

Outside North America and Australia
        Blackwell Scientific Publications Ltd.
        Osney Mead
        Oxford OX2 0EL
        England

Copyright © 1984, Blackwell Scientific Publications, Inc.

7th Printing 1995

Library of Congress Cataloging in Publication Data

Main entry under title:

Respiratory therapy competency evaluation manual.
1. Respiratory therapy — Handbooks, manuals, etc.
I. Scanlan, Craig D., 1947-
[DNLM: 1. Respiratory therapy. WB 342 R4339]
RC735.I5R48   1984   615.8'36   83-15889
ISBN 0-86542-015-7

CONTENTS

PREFACE

Over the last two decades, respiratory therapy has evolved from a technical support service of limited scope into a sophisticated discipline requiring the complex skills and behaviors characteristic of a true profession. This rapid evolution has placed extraordinary burdens on the profession's educational system, particularly on its role in providing assurances of the competency of its graduate practitioners.

No aspect of professional education is more important to its success in fulfilling this role than that of student evaluation. Unfortunately, the time, effort, and costs incurred in the development and implementation of a comprehensive system that is capable of objectively evaluating and documenting a complex repertoire of knowledge, skills and behaviors exceed the capacity of most programs. In the authors' experience, efforts to achieve this end are, more often than not, fragmentary, lacking in methodological rigor, and, consequently, of little practical utility.

This manual represents an ambitious attempt to overcome such limitations. When conscientiously applied and (where necessary) appropriately modified, it provides instructor and student alike with reliable and valid means to facilitate the development, refinement, evaluation, and documentation of clinical competency.

Over five years in planning, the manual has undergone extensive testing and successful trial utilization in hospital, community college, and university-based educational programs at both the technician and therapist levels. As a result, the methods and procedures described herein are capable of accommodating both the differences in educational settings and the inherent diversity of curriculum designs and grading systems found among the nation's respiratory therapy programs. Moreover, although other assessment tools are commercially available, this manual represents the only system specifically designed to integrate clinical knowledge, technical skills, and professional behavior within a single evaluative framework. This combination of flexibility and comprehensiveness should enhance both the utility of the manual and, ultimately, its impact upon program quality. To the extent that such goals are achieved, the authors' best intents will be realized.

Format

The manual consists of four major parts: Overview, Proficiency Evaluations, Behavioral Rating Scales, and Summary Records.

The Overview provides a brief orientation to the concepts underlying the assessment of clinical competency and describes the general methods and procedures governing the use of the manual. As are the other components of the manual, the Overview is addressed to the student rather than to the instructor or evaluator. This approach is based upon both our educational philosophy and the recognition that the manual is as much a student learning resource as an evaluative tool for the educator. It is for this reason that detailed instructions on how to use the manual for assessment and decision making are provided in a separate instructor's guide.

The Proficiency Evaluations section provides 40 procedural checklists for assessing students' performance of those technical skills most commonly required of the competent clinical practitioner. Selection of the specific skills included in this section was based upon both an analysis of contemporary expectations for entry-level practice and a review of the current curriculum standards for accreditation.

Unique to this evaluation system is the incorporation of an assessment of clinical knowledge as an integral component of each proficiency evaluation. The inclusion of this component follows from our conviction that technical proficiency consists of both applied knowledge and procedural skills, and that the transfer of such knowledge to the reality of clinical practice is an essential element of clinical competence.

The Behavioral Rating Scales section provides a complementary focus to the evaluation methods just described. It is the authors' firm belief that competency in the delivery of safe and effective respiratory care demands more of the practitioner than just clinical knowledge and procedural skills. In fact, more often than not, an individual's personal attributes and behavior alone separate professional practice from simple fulfillment of technical requirements. The behavioral rating scales provide the means necessary to both assist students in developing appropriate professional behaviors and evaluate their attainment. Moreover, the rating scales incorporate a mechanism whereby the achievement of technical proficiency and the demonstration of professional behavior can be integrated within a single decision-making framework. We firmly believe that it is only by integrating the evaluation of these domains of competence that valid judgments of students' clinical progress and achievement can be confidently drawn.

The Summary Records section provides the means necessary to monitor and document student progress and maintain a record, where appropriate, of both laboratory and clinical activity. With the achievement of clinical competence representing a cumulative process occurring over time, and with student activity varying according to schedules and assignments, such records facilitate administration of the evaluation system and, ultimately, contribute to its successful implementation.

Limitations

Although comprehensive in scope and flexible in design, this manual cannot be expected to serve all purposes of all users in all settings. Successful integration of its methods and procedures into an educational curriculum, therefore, requires a knowledge of its limitations.

First and foremost among these limitations is the recognition that a clinical evaluation system is only as good as the people who administer and implement it. Quality assessment tools and procedures are no substitute for skilled and knowledgeable instructors, supervisors, and evaluators. Successful utilization of this manual requires that all users be familiar with its contents and that those directly responsible for student evaluation be thoroughly trained in the application of those contents. Suggestions for evaluator training are provided in the instructor's guide.

Purists will find that many procedural descriptions do not coincide exactly with local, regional, or (where available) national standards for performance of specific technical skills. This is due, in part, to the need to provide clinically relevant and generic descriptions of performance that are applicable in a wide variety of settings. Although provisions have been made to accommodate differences in performance expectations according to venue, total agreement cannot (and will not) be realized until national standards are established for all technical skills. The authors hope that this manual will contribute to that end.

Lastly, as in any complex human endeavor, mistakes cannot be totally avoided. Although every attempt was made to ensure perfection in the manual's presentation, we acknowledge and assume responsibility for any unforeseen errors in its content or design. Users who accept the possibility of error will hopefully not be inconvenienced by its occurrence; we do however ask that, where evident, such problems be brought to our attention. Only in this manner can we continually refine and improve the usefulness of the manual for the respiratory therapy education community it was designed to serve.

ACKNOWLEDGMENTS

The authors are indebted to many individuals for their input and guidance in the planning, development, and completion of this manual. Without their efforts, the authors' best intents could never have been realized.

Christopher Tino, B.S., RRT, and Diane Delsardo, Ed.M., RRT, formerly Directors of Clinical Education in the Respiratory Therapy Program at Bookdale Community College, Lincroft, New Jersey, were instrumental in both the initial development of the prototype manual and its subsequent refinement. Their extensive clinical experience and educational expertise contributed much to the final product.

Laura B. Wetherell, B.S., RRT, Director of Clinical Education in the Respiratory Therapy Program at Ferris State College, Big Rapids, Michigan, assisted in the expanded trial application of the prototype manual and helped develop and refine many of the proficiency evaluations included in the final version. Likewise, Lillian Davis, R.N., RRT, Program Director, and William Arnold, RRT, Director of Clinical Education, both of the Massachusetts General Hospital School of Respiratory Therapy, contributed to the review and evaluation of the revised version of the manual.

The authors are also grateful for the clerical assistance and organizational expertise of Carolyn Davis, Secretary of the Department of Health Education, Evaluation and Research, School of Health Related Professions, University of Medicine and Dentistry of New Jersey. Without her efforts, the final manuscript would still by relegated to what must have been scores of yellow pads.

Lastly, the authors owe a large debt to the hundreds of students and (now) competent practitioners whose tireless efforts in applying and demonstrating their knowledge and skills both created the need and provided the basis for developing and testing the manual's contents. Their patience, support, and critical input throughout the trial stages of the manual's development proved invaluable and will certainly facilitate the progress of current and future students toward the goal of competency attainment. It is to these students—past, present, and future—that we dedicate this manual.

Additional copies of the evaluation forms found in this manual are available. For further information, please write Craig Associates, P.O. Box 8531, Red Bank, New Jersey 07701.

OVERVIEW
ORIENTATION OF THE MANUAL

Professional Education

For most of you, enrollment in a respiratory therapy program represents your first exposure to professional education. Professional education differs from other modes of learning mainly in the nature and level of expectations it sets. Like other modes of education, professional education requires that you develop and master a body of specialized knowledge. Professional education is unique, however, in that it requires the student to skillfully apply that knowledge in practical settings. Moreover, professional education establishes general expectations regarding personal attributes and behaviors that it deems necessary for the effective application of the skills constituting its curriculum.

Professional Competence

Professional competence, then, develops from a combination of the knowledge, skills, and behaviors necessary for the safe and effective delivery of professional services. A competent practitioner is one who has mastered this complex mix of attributes. Obviously, the exact combination that fosters success varies according to the nature and level of one's professional responsibilities. For example, a respiratory therapy practitioner who assumes responsibilities for diagnostic testing in a pulmonary function laboratory is not judged by the same criteria as one who specializes in the critical care of newborn infants. Fortunately, however, most professionals can agree upon what constitutes the basic attributes or competencies necessary for entry into a specific discipline. Naturally, such competencies provide the basis for both the credentialing and educational systems.

Competency-Based Education

Competency-based education employs those mechanisms necessary to ensure that students develop the knowledge, skills, and behaviors expected of the entry-level practitioner. Generally this goal requires a clear specification of performance expectations and a method to evaluate student achievement according to those expectations.

Evaluating Competency Achievement

Evaluating students' achievement of competency is no small task. As we have discussed, professional competence represents a complex combination of attributes, even at the level of entry into a field. As a result, no single method of evaluation can be expected to suffice. Moreover, since most elements of professional competence involve performance in practical settings, most evaluation methods must, of necessity, be based upon the direct observation of that performance. Lastly, since professional competence is developed over time and is cumulatively built upon increasingly complex types of performance, the evaluation of progress requires frequent assessment.

What does this all imply for you, the student? Quite simply, it means that your progress toward achieving the competencies required of the entry-level respiratory therapy practitioner will be frequently evaluated through the direct scrutiny of your instructors/evaluators and by a variety of assessment methods.

An Evaluation System

An evaluation system consists of an orderly combination of methods and procedures designed to assist instructor and student alike in the teaching, learning, evaluation, and documentation of the individual's progress toward achievement of professional competency. To fulfill these multiple purposes, such a system must provide clear and detailed descriptions of performance expectations and specify the standards, conditions, and procedures whereby such performance will be judged. This manual represents one such system.

PURPOSES AND USE OF THE MANUAL

Purposes

This manual was designed to serve as both a learning resource and evaluation tool. As a learning resource, you will find it an invaluable companion as you develop your skills and practice their application. As an evaluation tool, you and your instructors will use it to determine your readiness for and assess your ability to deliver safe and effective respiratory care. For these reasons, the manual should be kept available whenever and wherever you are involved in developing or applying your clinical skills.

Use

The use of this manual (as well as its availability) will, of course, be governed by your program faculty. Because the manual has been designed for application in a variety of educational settings, provisions have been made for your instructors to tailor its use to the specific needs of your program and its curriculum. For this reason, it is essential that you pay careful attention to any additional instructions and guidelines provided by your program faculty for the manual's use.

ORGANIZATION OF THE MANUAL

Three major sections follow this overview: Proficiency Evaluations, Behavioral Rating Scales, and Summary Records. A general knowledge of the contents of each section will help you understand how best to utilize the manual and exactly what to expect as you progress toward clinical competency. Detailed discussion of the applicable methods and procedures can be found at the beginning of each section.

Proficiency Evaluations (Section I)

This section constitutes the bulk of the manual and consists of descriptions of the numerous technical procedures commonly required of the respiratory therapy practitioner. Each procedural description consists of two components: (1) an evaluation checklist, and (2) procedural specifications.

The evaluation checklist, or Proficiency Evaluation Form, is an abbreviated, step-by-step listing of the actions required to properly execute a given procedure. Used by a trained evaluator, it provides the mechanism for recording and assessing your performance on that skill. It additionally furnishes the means to specify the pertinent condition(s) under which the evaluation took place and provides a method for rating your technical knowledge of the procedure. Lastly, the Proficiency Evaluation Form provides a record of the evaluator's overall judgment of your performance and evidence (by signature) of its review by appropriate personnel, including yourself.

Procedural specifications follow each Proficiency Evaluation Form. Procedural specifications elaborate on the procedural checklists, providing precise descriptions of performance expectations and requisite clinical knowledge. As such, the procedural specifications merit your careful attention, particularly in the development and practice phases of your learning. Only by adherence to these specifications, after all, can you expect to properly apply the skill and eventually demonstrate competence in its performance.

Behavioral Rating Scales (Section II)

This section consists of two forms of a multiattribute scale that simultaneously sets specific standards regarding your clinical behavior and provides a mechanism for assessing the extent to which such behavior is actually exhibited in the clinical component of your education.

Each form of the scale provides evaluators with the opportunity to rate your behavior according to the degree to which specific attributes are evidenced in your overall clinical performance. The "short form" or formative version of the scale has been designed to provide you with frequent qualitative feedback useful in developing and improving your clinical performance. Although its use may vary according to the specifications of your instructor(s), outcomes derived from the application of the formative rating scale are usually not employed for grading purposes. The "long form" or <u>summative</u> version of the scale provides more detailed specifications of each behavioral attribute and requires more explicit documentation to support their rating. As its name implies, the summative rating scale is usually employed as a tool in reaching final judgments of the quality of your overall clinical performance. These estimations are commonly used in determining your clinical grade.

From the student perspective, it is crucial that you have a clear understanding of these expectations (or modifications thereof) and continually strive to demonstrate behaviors consistent with the attributes described. Moreover, it is incumbent upon students to ensure that any evidence cited in support of evaluators' ratings be timely, relevant, and accurate. As with the Proficiency Evaluation Form, the opportunity is provided for students to review, comment, and confirm (by signature) evaluators' observations and conclusions.

Summary Records (Section III)

This section consists of five forms designed to facilitate documentation of your clinical learning activities and monitor your progress toward the achievement of clinical competency: (1) the Cumulative Proficiency Record, (2) the Proficiency Assignment Form, (3) the Summary Evaluation and Recommendation Form, (4) the Clinical Log Form, and (5) the Laboratory Activity and Attendance Record.

The <u>Cumulative Proficiency Record</u> provides a mechanism to document the achievement of proficiency in each of the technical skills included in Section I of this manual. In most programs, instructors and/or evaluators will maintain a duplicate Cumulative Proficiency Record on each student. Your instructor(s) will provide detailed instructions on how entries will be made and the Cumulative Proficiency Record maintained. Regardless of the procedures employed, it is essential that you keep an accurate record of your cumulative development of skills. Details on how to use this record for this purpose are provided in Section III.

The <u>Proficiency Assignment Form</u> provides a mechanism to specify the assignment of required proficiency evaluations by clinical site or rotation. Under most circumstances, your instructors will specify where or when you must undergo specific proficiency evaluations of your technical skills. Normally you are responsible for listing these assignments on this form and, ultimately, completing the assigned evaluations at the site or during the time designated.

The <u>Summary Evaluation and Recommendation Form</u> will normally be used by your instructors to combine outcomes derived from the proficiency evaluations (Section I) and the summary form of the Behavioral Rating Scale into an individualized "status" recommendation. It is included here so that you will be familiar with its format and the range of recommendations that can be formulated by your instructors. Details on how it will be applied in your specific program will be provided by your faculty.

The Clinical Log Form represents a suggested format for student recording of clinical activity. It is designed to provide documentation of procedures performed, observational learning, and physician contact. Although, as with the other summary records, its application will be based upon specifications provided by your instructors, it will normally be your responsibility to record and maintain as accurate and complete a description of your clinical activity as they deem necessary.

Similar in intent to the Clinical Log Form, the Laboratory Activity and Attendance Record provides a recommended format to briefly record your activities and document your attendance in the respiratory therapy learning laboratory. Since laboratory scheduling and assignments vary according to the nature of your program and its curriculum, guidelines on the use of this summary record will be provided by your instructors.

TOWARDS COMPETENCY ACHIEVEMENT

The methods and procedures described here have been designed to assist you and your instructors in developing, verifying, and documenting your achievement of the complex combination of knowledge, skills, and behaviors characterizing the competent respiratory therapy practitioner. Although the manual can facilitate your progress toward that end, it cannot guarantee it. No evaluation system, no matter how well designed, can substitute for the continuing and conscientious efforts of a highly motivated learner. As in any other meaningful endeavor, success in attaining clinical competency is ultimately dependent upon both your dedication to that goal and your perseverance in its pursuit. The road is long and arduous, but the rewards of achievement are substantial and, we believe, the journey is worthwhile.

I. PROFICIENCY EVALUATIONS

INTRODUCTION

A proficiency evaluation involves a short (10-30 minute) demonstration by a student of his or her competency in the performance of a specific respiratory care skill. The methods and procedures for assessing 40 of the most common technical skills required of the respiratory therapy practitioner are included in this section.

Setting

A proficiency evaluation may take place in the respiratory therapy laboratory, in the hospital or clinic, or in other locations designated by your instructors.

Laboratory. When required, many proficiency evaluations may be conducted in your learning laboratory. The purpose of evaluating your proficiency in this setting is usually to ensure that you have the knowledge and skills necessary to subsequently perform the procedure under direct supervision in the real world of the clinic or hospital. Such assessments of your proficiency, conducted under controlled or simulated conditions, are often referred to as "preclinical" or "readiness" evaluations. The extent to which you undergo preclinical evaluation will be determined by your faculty.

Alternatively, the laboratory setting may be used to assess your performance of skills that are otherwise difficult or impossible to effectively evaluate in the clinic. This type of proficiency evaluation is commonly employed when your instructors want you to demonstrate skill in the application of equipment or procedures not available in the clinic, or when performance of a particular procedure is so potentially hazardous as to preclude its real application by a neophyte.

Regardless of the purpose for which laboratory proficiency evaluations are conducted, it is essential that you understand both the advantages and limitations of this setting.

The major advantage of laboratory-based proficiency evaluations is the standardization or control of the conditions under which you are assessed. For the evaluator, controlled conditions increase the reliability with which judgments of student performance can be made. For the student, controlled conditions mean that all elements of the tested performance can be anticipated. Knowing that expectations have been clearly set and that conditions have been standardized should help allay your anxieties over the direct observation of your performance and focus your attention on the task at hand, i.e., demonstrating competency in carrying out the procedure being assessed.

As you might already expect, this major advantage of laboratory proficiency evaluation is also its most significant limitation. Although evaluation of your ability to perform technical skills in the laboratory may simulate many of the conditions encountered in the clinic, the key ingredient, i.e., a patient receiving respiratory care, is missing. Since many elements related to the application of skills to actual patients cannot be readily assessed in the laboratory, proficiency evaluation in this setting must limit its emphasis to the technical and equipment-related aspects of the task at hand.

Clinic.   Whereas laboratory evaluation is normally used to determine your readiness to subsequently apply skills in a practice setting, clinic evaluation is necessarily employed to confirm your ability to perform procedures on a variety of patients and/or under less controlled circumstances.

Clearly, the advantage of clinical proficiency evaluation lies in the reality of the test conditions. In terms of developing professional competency, no substitute exists for "hands-on" application of skills under knowledgeable guidance and supervision. Moreover, confirming competency achievement is generally impossible without directly observing performance under the diversity of conditions and in the variety of circumstances characterizing the clinical experience.

Although such diversity is both necessary and desirable, it tends to compound the difficulties encountered in evaluating your proficiency in applying technical skills. Lacking the standardized conditions characterizing the laboratory, the clinical setting is fraught with unanticipated events and consequences. The uncooperative patient, the untoward response to treatment, the mechanical failure of equipment—these are but a few of the common occurrences encountered by practitioners in fulfilling their daily responsibilities. That such events are commonly encountered by practitioners is, of course, all the more reason for ensuring that you gain equivalent exposure and that your ability to react and effectively deal with varying conditions be evaluated and confirmed. In the absence of such exposure and of a means to assess its impact, one's scope of competency is limited to the rote performance of simple tasks.

In order to overcome such limitations and ensure that your abilities are assessed under varying circumstances, the procedural specifications accompanying each Proficiency Evaluation Form provide options for both the conditions under which evaluation will occur and the nature of the equipment utilized in performance of each skill. Because expectations regarding these performance variables differ among programs, provisions have been made for your instructors to specify which conditions and which equipment apply to your proficiency evaluation.

The setting, conditions, and equipment specifications are normally recorded by your evaluator on the Proficiency Evaluation Form and provide the general framework for the actual evaluation activity.

Methods and Procedures

Proficiency evaluations are normally conducted by your instructors or their designees. Regardless of the setting, proficiency evaluations will usually consist of two parts: (1) performance of the procedure itself and (2) a short oral question and answer period.

Performance assessment. Performance of the procedure itself is assessed by observing you as you prepare for, implement, and complete the task at hand. During observation, the evaluator compares your performance to the steps delineated on the Proficiency Evaluation Form and described in the procedural specifications accompanying each form.

When a step in the procedure is performed correctly, i.e., according to the description of satisfactory performance provided in the procedural specifications, the evaluator will check the box labeled "Satisfactory." Under most circumstances, an overall evaluation of satisfactory on the skill being assessed will require that your performance be error-free, i.e., that all steps be judged as correctly performed.

Errors in performing a technical skill can be categorized as <u>either errors of commission</u> or <u>errors of omission</u>. You commit an <u>error of commission</u> when you perform an applicable step but make a procedural mistake, i.e., you fail to meet the criteria for satisfactory performance described in the procedural specifications. You commit an error of omission when you leave out a step that should have been performed.

Provision has been made on the Proficiency Evaluation Forms for evaluators to differentiate between these two categories of errors. Should you commit an error of commission in performance of a particular step, the evaluator will check the corresponding box labeled "Unsatisfactory." On the other hand, should you leave out a required step, the evaluator will check the "Not Observed" box pertaining to the element of the procedure.

Errors of both commission and omission may be further categorized according to their importance. A <u>critical error</u> will normally be defined by your instructors as one that <u>could either</u> (1) endanger the patient or (2) result in a less than satisfactory procedural outcome. A <u>minor error</u>, on the other hand, represents a deviation from optimum performance that, although technically incorrect, would normally not affect the outcome of the procedure or the patient's well-being. Because the magnitude of an error and its impact varies according to the conditions under which a procedure is performed, it is generally impossible to prespecify which steps can result in critical errors and which steps are limited to minor errors. Normally, prior to a specific proficiency evaluation session, your evaluator will designate the potential for critical errors.

Review of the format of the Proficiency Evaluation Form will indicate the presence of a fourth category of evaluator response to your performance, i.e., "Not Applicable." This response is reserved for those situations in which, according to the judgment of your evaluator, the step in question did not apply under the conditions present at the time of assessment. Such a response has been provided to accommodate changes necessitated by the circumstances and/or variations in local or regional interpretation of optimum best practice. Unlike the Unsatisfactory or Not Observed response, the Not Applicable category implies no negative consequences.

In addition to evaluating your proficiency in the step-by-step performance of skills, your instructors may require, for some procedures, that specific results or outcomes be achieved. A good example of the need to include outcome assessment as a component of some proficiency evaluations is the skill of measuring a patient's blood pressure. Certainly, precise adherence to the steps in implementing this procedure is a necessary precondition for obtaining accurate results, i.e., the patient's blood pressure. It is, however, possible to follow the procedure to the letter (at least according to what is observable) and still obtain erroneous results. For this reason, the procedural specifications component of those skills for which a tangible result is expected include a delineation of "Outcome Criteria." Achievement of these additional criteria, where applicable, is normally indicated in the outcome criteria section of the Proficiency Evaluation Form. If the desired results are not achieved, your evaluator will indicate which criteria were not met or, alternatively, whether constraints beyond your control prevented their attainment.

Oral review. Following completion of the procedure itself, your evaluator will normally ask you a short series of standardized questions related to the specific skill being evaluated. The intent of these questions is to confirm your knowledge of the essential elements of the task at hand. Oral review questions for each skill are included in the procedural specifications component of the applicable proficiency evaluation.

After completion of the oral review questions, your evaluator will rate your comprehension of the procedure on the five-point scale provided on the Proficiency Evaluation Form. Although expectations may differ among programs, most instructors will require that you demonstrate at least an "adequate" comprehension of the key concepts related to the procedure being assessed. Depending upon the guidelines established by your program personnel, failure to demonstrate the appropriate level of knowledge for a given procedure could contribute to a less than satisfactory overall evaluation, even if you demonstrated proficiency in the actual application of the skill. Detailed instructions on how the oral review component of your proficiency evaluations will be integrated into the summary evaluation of your performance will be provided by your program faculty.

Summary performance evaluation. After completion of the procedural demonstration and (where required) the oral review, your evaluator will provide a summary judgment of your overall proficiency in performing the task at hand. At this stage of the decision-making process, only one of two summary judgments can be drawn. Your overall performance will be judged as either satisfactory or unsatisfactory.

Recommendations based upon this summary judgment depend upon the setting in which you were evaluated. In the laboratory setting, a satisfactory summary evaluation of your proficiency in performing a specific skill will usually result in a recommendation that you go on to apply the skill, under supervision, in the clinic. Alternatively, an unsatisfactory summary judgment stemming from performance deficiencies observed in this setting will normally result in a recommendation that you spend additional laboratory time on practicing and remediating the problems identified. Such a recommendation may, according to your program's procedures, require that you undergo a subsequent laboratory re-evaluation before proceeding to direct clinical application.

In the clinical setting, a satisfactory summary evaluation will usually result in a recommendation that you be allowed to apply and refine that particular skill under less direct supervision. Recommendations stemming from an unsatisfactory summary evaluation of your proficiency in the clinical setting, unlike that described for the laboratory, may take one of two alternate forms. When the unsatisfactory rating is based on your commitment of critical errors, a complete re-evaluation of your clinical proficiency is usually called for. When, on the other hand, the judgment of unsatisfactory performance is based on minor and easily rectifiable errors, your evaluator will probably recommend that you be reassessed only in regard to those components of the procedure on which your performance was judged less than optimum. In either case (and in either setting) your evaluator will reiterate the errors or deficiencies encountered and, where time allows, provide guidance as to how best to correct your problem areas. Should the deficiencies noted in the clinical setting be so significant as to threaten the well-being of the patient, your evaluator may suggest or require that you go back to the laboratory prior to attempting further clinical evaluation.

Where necessary or appropriate, evaluators may provide amplification or clarification on their observations in the section of the Proficiency Evaluation Form labeled "Additional Comments."

Lastly, your evaluator will normally document, in abbreviated form, the overall outcome of each proficiency evaluation in the appropriate box of the Cumulative Proficiency Record, which is found in Section III of this manual.

Student Responsibilities

Successful application of the proficiency evaluation component of this manual is largely dependent on the student's fulfillment of several key responsibilities. Foremost among these responsibilities are pre-evaluation preparation and postevaluation record keeping.

Preparation. No aspect of the proficiency evaluation procedure is more critical to your successful achievement than preliminary preparation. Ideally, the preparatory stage of proficiency evaluation should consist of three phases: (1) observation, (2) practice, and (3) trial evaluation.

The observation phase usually coincides with demonstrations of technical skills provided by your instructors or their designees. During a demonstration, your instructor will normally review the key aspects of a given skill and provide a step-by-step example of the actions required to properly execute the procedure. During a demonstration, it is essential that you pay careful attention to your instructor's explanations and note, where applicable, special instructions or guidelines, particularly those that relate to your program faculty's expectations regarding the conditions or equipment specifications applicable to your evaluation. In some settings, the demonstration will be supplemented (or supplanted) with videotaped examples of procedural performance.

The practice phase of proficiency evaluation is, of course, the most important of all student preparatory responsibilities. Only by practicing the various elements of a procedure can you later expect to demonstrate proficiency in its performance. During this phase, it is essential that you carefully review and adhere to the descriptions of satisfactory performance provided in the procedural specifications component of the applicable proficiency evaluation.* Where necessary or desirable, skills requiring patient interaction should be practiced on peers. Such peer practice must, of course, be limited to those skills that present minimal hazards to the recipient.

Where time permits and conditions allow, your practice of a particular skill should be followed by a trial evaluation. Such dry runs can alert you to details that might otherwise be overlooked and can significantly bolster your confidence in undergoing subsequent formal evaluation. Trial evaluation can commonly take one or more of three forms: (1) self-assessment, (2) peer assessment, and (3) observational assessment.

As the name implies, trial evaluation by self-assessment simply requires that you go through the procedure yourself, carefully comparing your actions to the pre-established expectations provided in the procedural specifications component of the applicable proficiency evaluation. Although useful, self-assessment can be misleading and should be reserved for those instances in which other methods of trial evaluation cannot be employed.

Peer assessment is the most effective method of trial evaluation. This is based, in part, on research indicating that students are often more critical of each others' performance than are their own instructors! In addition to the close scrutiny usually provided by fellow students, trial evaluation by peers provides a necessary external reference to your performance, a reference that is not obtainable by self-assessment methods. Such a perspective often reveals problem areas not otherwise evident to the learner and can increase the likelihood of your success on subsequent formal evaluations.

Observational assessment represents a third method of trial evaluation. It differs from self- and peer assessment in that others' performance, rather than your own, provides the object of evaluation. Placing yourself in the position of evaluator provides unique insight into the performance expectations required in carrying out a particular skill and can represent a valuable learning experience. When you serve as the external observer conducting an evaluation of a peer, you are, of course, participating in preparation through observational assessment. Alternatively, your instructors may provide you

---

*Those procedural steps that are common to most respiratory care skills are grouped together in the Common Performance Elements component of this section.

with the opportunity to observe and assess the performance of others on videotape. This mode of observational assessment is particularly valuable as a preparatory method when you can compare your assessment to that previously determined by your instructors. Regardless of the method chosen, however, observational assessment techniques should be considered only as supplements to the more conventional methods of trial evaluation.

Depending on the instructions provided by your faculty, preparation for proficiency evaluation may also require review of the requisite knowledge pertaining to the skill being assessed. Such review is best accomplished by using the oral review questions provided in the procedural specifications as a guide to applicable readings, class notes, and handouts. Following the review of such resource material, practice question and answer sessions with other students can provide the assurances necessary to successfully complete this component of the formal proficiency evaluation.

Record keeping. Following each proficiency evaluation, you should review the documentation with your evaluator and ensure that all appropriate entries are complete and accurate. Failure to do so can result in confusion regarding your status or unnecessarily delay your progress toward competency achievement.

COMMON PERFORMANCE ELEMENTS

COMMON PERFORMANCE ELEMENTS

Common Performance Elements are frequently occurring steps common to many of the procedures performed by a respiratory care practitioner. Provided below is a list of these recurrent elements or steps (as they appear on each Proficiency Evaluation Form) and a description of exactly what constitutes satisfactory performance for that step. An asterisk (*) appears next to those performance descriptions that are, by themselves, discrete procedures evaluated by proficiency demonstration.

Procedural Element (Step)	Description of Satisfactory Performance
Washes hands*	Refer to applicable proficiency evaluation
Selects, gathers, and assembles appropriate equipment	Obtains equipment and accessories necessary to perform the procedure Preassembles components properly, avoiding contamination

Verifies, interprets, and evaluates physician's order	Ensures that requisition matches order
	Ensures that order is complete
	Reviews pertinent data (medical records)*
	Notes special considerations, including:
	  a. nonroutine characteristics of treatment
	  b. information related to type, dosage of medication
	  c. special instructions or precautions
	  d. potential hazards or contraindications of therapy or procedure

Identifies patient, self, and department	Confirms patient identity by:
	  a. checking room number and patient's name on door or bed
	  b. addressing patient by name
	  c. checking patient identity band
	Introduces self by name and department

Explains procedure and confirms patient understanding	Informs patient of procedure to be performed
	Explains procedure by describing:
	  a. why it is to be performed
	  b. how it is to be performed
	  c. how frequently it will be performed
	  d. importance of patient cooperation
	Asks patient if there are any questions regarding procedures
	Provides answers that are accurate and appropriate to patient's level of understanding

Maintains/processes equipment	Discards disposable equipment Replaces nondisposable equipment according to departmental schedule Removes equipment not in use from room OR unplugs, covers, and stores equipment away from patient's bedside Isolates contaminated equipment Checks in-use equipment as scheduled Forwards and prepares dirty equipment for processing

Records pertinent data in chart and departmental records	Records the following data (where applicable):
	  a. date
	  b. time (length of therapy/procedure
	  c. treatment given (including medication dosage)
	  d. patient assessment (subjective/objective)
	  e. patient tolerance/adverse reactions
	  f. patient complaints
	  g. any other pertinent observations or data

Records pertinent data in chart and departmental records (continued)	Charts in inks (correct color) Crosses through errors and signifies as such Does not skip lines Signs entry with name, student designation Has entry verified by supervisor
Notifies appropriate personnel	Informs nurse and/or physician of: a. patient requests b. patient complaints c. untoward response to therapy d. other pertinent observations of patient

BASIC SKILLS

STUDENT:	DATE:

PROCEDURE (TASK): VITAL SIGNS

	SATISFACTORY	UNSATISFACTORY	NOT OBSERVED	NOT APPLICABLE
SETTING: ☐ LABORATORY ☐ OTHER: (SPECIFY) ☐ CLINIC				
CONDITIONS (DESCRIBE)				
EQUIPMENT UTILIZED:				
STEPS IN PROCEDURE OR TASK:				
PATIENT PREPARATION				
1. Washes hands				
2. Checks chart (graphic history, vital signs)				
3. Identifies patient, self, and department				
4. Explains procedure and confirms patient understanding				
IMPLEMENTATION				
5. Positions patient (provides for privacy, comfort)				
6. Palpates appropriate artery				
7. Counts pulsations for specified time				
8. Notes rate, force, and rythmicity of beats				
9. Observes rate, depth, and rythmicity of respirations				
10. Repositions patient				
11. Reassures patient				
FOLLOW-UP				
12. Records pertinent data in chart and departmental records				
13. Notifies appropriate personnel				

STUDENT'S COMPREHENSION OF PROCEDURE (SELECT ONE ONLY)

The student demonstrates comprehensive knowledge of basic and advanced concepts beyond requirements of procedure	
The student demonstrates above average understanding of basic concepts applicable to the skill demonstrated	
The student demonstrates adequate knowledge of the essential elements of the task performed	
The student shows limited understanding of essential concepts related to the procedure	
The student has inadequate knowledge of even the basic concepts related to the task at hand	

OUTCOME CRITERIA (WHERE APPLICABLE)

☐ MET	SPECIFY CRITERIA NOT MET AND/OR PERTINENT CONSTRAINTS
☐ NOT MET	
☐ NOT APPL.	

ADDITIONAL COMMENTS

Include errors of omission or commission; if clinical therapeutic procedure emphasize communicative skills (verbal and non-verbal) and effectiveness of patient interaction:

SUMMARY PERFORMANCE EVALUATION AND RECOMMENDATIONS

SETTING	SATISFACTORY	UNSATISFACTORY	SPECIFY DEFICIENCIES
LABORATORY	☐ Can now perform skill under direct clinical supervision	☐ Requires additional laboratory practice	
CLINIC	☐ Ready for minimally supervised application and refinement	☐ Requires additional supervised clinical practice 　☐ Complete re-evaluation required 　☐ Re-evaluation·minor deficiencies only	

STUDENT:　　　　　　EVALUATOR:　　　　　FACULTY:

PROCEDURAL SPECIFICATIONS
VITAL SIGNS

I. Key Performance Elements

Procedural Element (Step)	Description of Satisfactory Performance
2. Checks chart (graphic history, vital signs)	Ascertains current patient status Locates and identifies most recent vital signs and trends
5. Positions patient (provides for privacy, comfort)	Draws curtain Places patient in semi-Fowler's position (or comfortable alternative)
6. Palpates appropriate artery	Selects radial artery (unless contraindicated) Places middle three finger-tips over artery Applies appropriate pressure
7. Counts pulsations for specified time	Counts beats for 60 seconds Uses watch to time interval
9. Observes rate, depth and rhythmicity of respirations	Observes chest excursions unobtrusively Maintains count for a minimum of 30 seconds Extends count if irregularities noted

II. Setting

The student is expected to demonstrate proficiency in the assessment of vital signs in the following setting: (check those that apply)

☐ Laboratory

☐ Clinic

☐ Other (specify)

_____

_____

III. Conditions

The student is expected to demonstrate proficiency in the assessment of vital signs under the following conditions: (check those that apply)

Patient Variables

☐ Simulated (peer)

☐ Infant

☐ Child

☐ Adult

Procedure Variables

☐ Radial pulse

☐ Brachial pulse

☐ Femoral pulse

☐ Carotid pulse

Other conditional specifications: _____

_____

_____

IV. Equipment

Not applicable

V. Outcome Criteria

Noted rate, force (depth), and rhythmicity of pulsations and respirations recorded in chart and departmental records must correspond to those concurrently determined by the evaluator.

VI. Oral Review Questions

1. What are the normal ranges of pulse rate and respirations for newborn infants? for 5 year old children? for male adults? for female adults?

2. What are some common causes for absent arterial pulsations? for weak pulsations? for irregularities in pulsations?

3. Define and identify some potential causes of the following:
   a. bradycardia
   b. tachycardia
   c. pulsus paradoxus
   d. pulsus altercans
   e. "bounding" pulse
   f. "thready" pulse

4. What other methods (other than palpation) can be used to measure heart rate?   What additional information can these provide?

5. Define and describe the observable manifestations and potential causes of the following respiratory patterns:
   a. eupnea
   b. tachypnea
   c. bradypnea
   d. hyperpnea
   e. hypopnea
   f. Biot's respirations
   g. Cheyne-Stokes respirations
   h. Kussmaul's respirations

STUDENT:	DATE:				

PROCEDURE (TASK): ARTERIAL BLOOD PRESSURE

SETTING: ☐ LABORATORY ☐ OTHER: (SPECIFY) ☐ CLINIC	SATISFACTORY	UNSATISFACTORY	NOT OBSERVED	NOT APPLICABLE
CONDITIONS (DESCRIBE)				
EQUIPMENT UTILIZED:				

STEPS IN PROCEDURE OR TASK:				
EQUIPMENT AND PATIENT PREPARATION				
1. Washes hands				
2. Selects, gathers, and assembles appropriate equipment				
3. Checks chart (graphic history, vital signs, contraindications)				
4. Identifies patient, self, and department				
5. Explains procedure and confirms patient understanding				
IMPLEMENTATION				
6. Positions patient				
7. Positions/secures cuff properly				
8. Adjusts stethoscope position				
9. Closes pump valve				
10. Inflates cuff				
11. Reassures patient				
12. Opens valve, releases pressure slowly				
13. Observes manometer/listens to pulse sounds				
14. Records systolic/diasystolic pressures				
15. Repeats procedure to confirm results				
16. Removes equipment from patient's arm				
17. Reassures patient (repositions if necessary)				
FOLLOW-UP				
18. Records readings on appropriate records				
19. Maintains/processes equipment				
20. Notifies appropriate personnel				

STUDENT'S COMPREHENSION OF PROCEDURE (SELECT ONE ONLY)

The student demonstrates comprehensive knowledge of basic and advanced concepts beyond requirements of procedure	
The student demonstrates above average understanding of basic concepts applicable to the skill demonstrated	
The student demonstrates adequate knowledge of the essential elements of the task performed	
The student shows limited understanding of essential concepts related to the procedure	
The student has inadequate knowledge of even the basic concepts related to the task at hand	

OUTCOME CRITERIA (WHERE APPLICABLE)

☐ MET	SPECIFY CRITERIA NOT MET AND/OR PERTINENT CONSTRAINTS
☐ NOT MET	
☐ NOT APPL.	

ADDITIONAL COMMENTS

Include errors of omission or commission; if clinical therapeutic procedure emphasize communicative skills (verbal and non-verbal) and effectiveness of patient interaction:

SUMMARY PERFORMANCE EVALUATION AND RECOMMENDATIONS

SETTING	SATISFACTORY	UNSATISFACTORY	SPECIFY DEFICIENCIES
LABORATORY	☐ Can now perform skill under direct clinical supervision	☐ Requires additional laboratory practice	

CLINIC	☐ Ready for minimally supervised application and refinement	☐ Requires additional supervised clinical practice
		  ☐ Complete re-evaluation required
		  ☐ Re-evaluation·minor deficiencies only	

STUDENT: EVALUATOR: FACULTY:

PROCEDURAL SPECIFICATIONS
ARTERIAL BLOOD PRESSURE

I. Key Performance Elements

Procedural Element (Step)	Description of Satisfactory Performance
2. Selects, gathers, and assembles appropriate equipment	Selects cuff 20% wider than diameter of limb Selects diaphragm-type stethoscope
3. Checks chart (graphic history, vital signs, contraindications)	Ascertain current patient status Locates and identifies most recent vital signs and trends Notes contraindications to cuff placement
6. Positions patient	Utilizes supine or semi-Fowler's position where possible Places arm in outstretched position
7. Positions/secures cuff properly	Places cuff so that lower edge is 2.5 cm above antecubital fossa for brachial pressure measurement Places rubber bag anteriorly
8. Adjusts stethoscope position	Palpates/locates artery Places stethoscope over artery
10. Inflates cuff	Increases cuff pressure 20 mmHg above disappearance of all audible sounds
13. Observes manometer/listens to pulse sounds	Ascertains appearance/disappearance of Korotkoff's sounds

II. Setting

The student is expected to demonstrate proficiency in the measurement of arterial blood pressure in the following settings: (check those that apply)

☐ Laboratory   ☐ Other (specify):

☐ Clinic

_____

_____

III. Conditions

The student is expected to demonstrate proficiency in the measurement of arterial blood pressure under the following conditions: (check those that apply)

Patient Variables   Procedure Variables

☐ Simulated (peer)   ☐ Brachial artery (arm)

☐ Infant   ☐ Popliteal artery (thigh)

☐ Child

☐ Adult

Other conditional specifications: _____

_____

_____

IV. Equipment

The student is expected to demonstrate proficiency in the measurement of arterial blood pressure using the following equipment: (check those that apply)

☐ Aneroid sphygmomanometer

☐ Mercurial sphygmomanometer

☐ Other (specify): _____

_____

V. Outcome Criteria

Measured systolic, diastolic, and calculated pulse pressures must correspond to those concurrently determined by the evaluator (degree of accuracy = ± 5%)

VI. Oral Review Questions

1. What are the major physiological determinants of arterial blood pressure (systolic, diastolic)?

2. Identify 6–8 physiological or pathological factors which can alter normal blood pressure.

3. What are the normal ranges of brachial blood pressure (systolic/diastolic) for newborn infants? for young children? for young adults?

4. What are the major sources of error in blood pressure determinations?

5. What is the significance of the mean arterial pressure and how can it be estimated?

6. What is the significance of the pulse pressure? What is its normal value (adult)? What factors determine pulse pressure? What are the physiological causes for increased/decreased pulse pressure?

STUDENT:	DATE:

PROCEDURE (TASK): PATIENT POSITIONING

SETTING: ☐ LABORATORY ☐ OTHER: (SPECIFY) ☐ CLINIC	SATISFACTORY	UNSATISFACTORY	NOT OBSERVED	NOT APPLICABLE
CONDITIONS (DESCRIBE)				
EQUIPMENT UTILIZED:				

STEPS IN PROCEDURE OR TASK:				
EQUIPMENT AND PATIENT PREPARATION	▒	▒	▒	▒
1. Washes hands				
2. Selects and gathers appropriate equipment				
3. Checks chart for order/contraindications to positioning				
4. Identifies patient, self, and department				
5. Explains procedure and confirms patient understanding				
IMPLEMENTATION	▒	▒	▒	▒
6. Provides patient privacy				
7. Adjusts bed to working level				
8. Lowers siderails				
9. Removes supportive pillows				
10. Positions patient/bed				
11. Restores supportive aids				
12. Adjusts patient's body alignment				
13. Provides protection against pressure points				
14. Raises siderails				
FOLLOW-UP	▒	▒	▒	▒
15. Provides for patient's safety/comfort				
16. Rechecks alignment/support of patient				
17. Repositions as necessary (steps 5-14 above)				
18. Records change of position and patient observations				
19. Notifies appropriate personnel				

STUDENT'S COMPREHENSION OF PROCEDURE (SELECT ONE ONLY)

The student demonstrates comprehensive knowledge of basic and advanced concepts beyond requirements of procedure	
The student demonstrates above average understanding of basic concepts applicable to the skill demonstrated	
The student demonstrates adequate knowledge of the essential elements of the task performed	
The student shows limited understanding of essential concepts related to the procedure	
The student has inadequate knowledge of even the basic concepts related to the task at hand	

OUTCOME CRITERIA (WHERE APPLICABLE)

☐ MET	SPECIFY CRITERIA NOT MET AND/OR PERTINENT CONSTRAINTS
☐ NOT MET	
☐ NOT APPL.	

ADDITIONAL COMMENTS

Include errors of omission or commission; if clinical therapeutic procedure emphasize communicative skills (verbal and non-verbal) and effectiveness of patient interaction:

SUMMARY PERFORMANCE EVALUATION AND RECOMMENDATIONS

SETTING	SATISFACTORY	UNSATISFACTORY	SPECIFY DEFICIENCIES
LABORATORY	☐ Can now perform skill under direct clinical supervision	☐ Requires additional laboratory practice	
CLINIC	☐ Ready for minimally supervised application and refinement	☐ Requires additional supervised clinical practice ☐ Complete re-evaluation required ☐ Re-evaluation·minor deficiencies only	

STUDENT:	EVALUATOR:	FACULTY:

PROCEDURAL SPECIFICATIONS
PATIENT POSITIONING

I. Key Performance Elements

Procedural Element (Step)	Description of Satisfactory Performance
3. Checks chart for order/ contraindications to positioning	Reviews chart (history, physical, progress notes, orders) to identify hazards/contraindications to position, to include: a. orthopnea b. high intracranial pressure c. hypotension d. decubiti
12. Adjusts patient's body alignment	Ensures patient's head, neck, and back are aligned Minimizes unnecessary flexion/ extension of muscles

II. Setting

The student is expected to demonstrate proficiency in the application of patient positioning techniques in the following settings: (check those that apply)

☐ Laboratory   ☐ Other (specify)

☐ Clinic

_____

_____

III. Conditions

The student is expected to demonstrate proficiency in the application of patient positioning techniques under the following conditions: (check those that apply)

Patient Variables   Procedure Variables

☐ Simulated (peer)   ☐ Supine position

☐ Infant   ☐ Prone position

☐ Child   ☐ Sim's position

☐ Adult   ☐ Fowler's position

                            ☐ Trendelenburg

Other conditional specifications: _____

_____

_____

IV. Equipment

The student is expected to demonstrate proficiency in the application of patient positioning techniques using the following
equipment: (check those that apply)

☐ Manually operated hospital bed

☐ Electrically operated hospital bed

☐ Standard residential bed (with adjuncts)

☐ Pediatric crib

☐ Other (specify) _____

_____

V. Outcome Criteria

Where possible, after positioning or repositioning, patient must
confirm comfort to evaluator. All safety considerations must be
met (siderails raised, etc.).

VI. Oral Review Questions

1. Changing a patient's position can help accomplish what desirable outcomes?

2. What is the physiological basis for Trendelenburg positions
   being contraindicated in the following situations:
   a. congestive heart failure?
   b. neurosurgery?
   c. chronic emphysema?

3. What effect does positional change have upon the distribution
   of gas within the lungs?

STUDENT:	DATE:

PROCEDURE (TASK): PATIENT ASSESSMENT

SETTING: ☐ LABORATORY ☐ OTHER: (SPECIFY)
☐ CLINIC

CONDITIONS (DESCRIBE)

EQUIPMENT UTILIZED:

STEPS IN PROCEDURE OR TASK:	SATISFACTORY	UNSATISFACTORY	NOT OBSERVED	NOT APPLICABLE
EQUIPMENT AND PATIENT PREPARATION				
1. Washes hands				
2. Selects, gathers, and assembles appropriate equipment				
3. Reviews pertinent chart information				
4. Identifies patient, self, and department				
5. Explains procedure and confirms patient understanding				
IMPLEMENTATION				
6. Positions patient (provides for privacy, comfort)				
7. Assesses patient's vital signs				
8. Inspects patient's thorax				
9. Palpates patient's thorax				
10. Percusses patient's thorax				
11. Auscultates patient's thorax				
12. Measures patient's ventilatory parameters				
13. Repositions patient, clothing, bedding				
14. Reassures patient				
FOLLOW-UP				
15. Maintains/processes equipment				
16. Records pertinent data in chart and departmental records				
17. Notifies appropriate personnel				

STUDENT'S COMPREHENSION OF PROCEDURE (SELECT ONE ONLY)

The student demonstrates comprehensive knowledge of basic and advanced concepts beyond requirements of procedure	
The student demonstrates above average understanding of basic concepts applicable to the skill demonstrated	
The student demonstrates adequate knowledge of the essential elements of the task performed	
The student shows limited understanding of essential concepts related to the procedure	
The student has inadequate knowledge of even the basic concepts related to the task at hand	

OUTCOME CRITERIA (WHERE APPLICABLE)

☐ MET	SPECIFY CRITERIA NOT MET AND/OR PERTINENT CONSTRAINTS
☐ NOT MET	
☐ NOT APPL.	

ADDITIONAL COMMENTS

Include errors of omission or commission; if clinical therapeutic procedure emphasize communicative skills (verbal and non-verbal) and effectiveness of patient interaction:

SUMMARY PERFORMANCE EVALUATION AND RECOMMENDATIONS

SETTING	SATISFACTORY	UNSATISFACTORY	SPECIFY DEFICIENCIES
LABORATORY	☐ Can now perform skill under direct clinical supervision	☐ Requires additional laboratory practice	
CLINIC	☐ Ready for minimally supervised application and refinement	☐ Requires additional supervised clinical practice ☐ Complete re-evaluation required ☐ Re-evaluation·minor deficiencies only	

STUDENT: EVALUATOR: FACULTY:

PROCEDURAL SPECIFICATIONS
PATIENT ASSESSMENT

I. Key Performance Elements

Procedural Element (Step)	Description of Satisfactory Performance
3. Reviews pertinent chart information	Checks history/physical records Checks progress notes Identifies any hazards/contraindications to assessment techniques
6. Positions patient (provides for privacy, comfort)	Draws curtain Places patient in Fowler's (sitting position) with support Removes necessary bedclothing, accommodates modesty
7. Assesses patient's vital signs	Refer to proficiency evaluations: VITAL SIGNS BLOOD PRESSURE
8. Inspects patient's thorax	Notes breathing pattern, frequency, inspiratory/expiratory ratio Identifies use of accessory muscles Assesses posture/shape of chest Identifies structural abnormalities
9. Palpates patient's thorax	Palpates trachea/notes position Palpates for vocal fremitus/notes abnormalities Determines lateral thoracic excursion Identifies/notes tissues/bony abnormalities

10. Percusses patient's thorax

Places distal phalanx of pleximeter in contact with thoracic wall

Taps pleximeter with tip of plexor finger sharply

Differentiates between areas of
   a. resonance
   b. hyperresonance
   c. dull notes
   d. flat notes

Determines presence of underlying organs

Determines vertical excusion of diaphragm

Identifies/notes tissue abnormalities

11. Auscultates patient's thorax

Warms stethoscope with hand

Positions diaphragm of stethoscope in rotation bisymmetrically throughout lung fields (posterior/anterior)

Distinguishes location and occurrence of adventitious breath sounds

12. Measures patient's ventilatory parameters

Refer to proficiency evaluations:
BEDSIDE VENTILATORY ASSESSMENT

II. Setting

The student is expected to demonstrate proficiency in patient assessment techniques in the following settings: (check those that apply)

☐ Laboratory

☐ Clinic

☐ Other (specify)

_____

_____

III. Conditions

The student is expected to demonstrate proficiency in patient assessment techniques under the following conditions: (check those that apply)

Patient Variables   Status Variables

☐   Simulated (peer)   ☐   No known abnormalities

☐   Infant   ☐   Abnormalities, unknown

☐   Child   ☐   Abnormalities, known

☐   Adult   (specify): _____

_____

_____

Other conditional specifications: _____

_____

_____

IV. Equipment

Applicable equipment is that pertaining to the related Proficiency Evaluations VITAL SIGNS, BLOOD PRESSURE, and BEDSIDE VENTILATORY ASSESSMENT.

V. Outcome Criteria

The student's description of findings resulting from inspection, palpation, percussion, and auscultation of the patient will correspond to those either noted concurrently by the evaluator, or (where findings are stable), those indicated in the most recent physical examination summary of the physician. In addition, measured values of vital signs, blood pressure, and ventilatory parameters will correspond to those measured concurrently by the evaluator (degree of accuracy ± 5%).

VI. Oral Review Questions

1. What are the "typical" findings on physical assessment (inspection, palpation, percussion, and auscultation) for each of the following conditions?
   a. chronic bronchitis
   b. emphysema
   c. asthma
   d. tension pneumothorax
   e. pneumonia (with consolidation)
   f. atelectasis
   g. congestive heart failure
   h. pulmonary edema
   i. pleural effusion

2. Relate the physical findings of the patient just assessed to the underlying pathophysiological disturbance characterizing his/her disease process.

STUDENT:		DATE:			

PROCEDURE (TASK): MEDICAL RECORDS					

	SATISFACTORY	UNSATISFACTORY	NOT OBSERVED	NOT APPLICABLE
SETTING: ☐ LABORATORY ☐ OTHER: (SPECIFY) ☐ CLINIC				
CONDITIONS (DESCRIBE)				
EQUIPMENT UTILIZED:				

STEPS IN PROCEDURE OR TASK:				
IMPLEMENTATION				
1. Identifies and locates patient chart				
2. Informs appropriate personnel of chart use/location				
3. Ascertains and summarizes				
a. age/admitting diagnosis				
b. drug allergies				
c. current medications				
d. pertinent medical history/physical condition				
e. present condition				
f. diagnostic studies in progress				
4. Determines most current respiratory therapy orders				
5. Explains rationale for ordered therapy				
6. Evaluates appropriateness of respiratory therapy orders				
7. Suggests alternative therapy/rationale				
8. Implements therapy				
9. Records objective/subjective evaluation of patient response to therapy				
10. Explains ethical/legal principles of medical record-keeping				
FOLLOW-UP				
11. Returns chart to proper location				
12. Informs appropriate personnel				

STUDENT'S COMPREHENSION OF PROCEDURE (SELECT ONE ONLY)

The student demonstrates comprehensive knowledge of basic and advanced concepts beyond requirements of procedure	
The student demonstrates above average understanding of basic concepts applicable to the skill demonstrated	
The student demonstrates adequate knowledge of the essential elements of the task performed	
The student shows limited understanding of essential concepts related to the procedure	
The student has inadequate knowledge of even the basic concepts related to the task at hand	

OUTCOME CRITERIA (WHERE APPLICABLE)

☐ MET	SPECIFY CRITERIA NOT MET AND/OR PERTINENT CONSTRAINTS
☐ NOT MET	
☐ NOT APPL.	

ADDITIONAL COMMENTS

Include errors of omission or commission; if clinical therapeutic procedure emphasize communicative skills (verbal and non-verbal) and effectiveness of patient interaction:

SUMMARY PERFORMANCE EVALUATION AND RECOMMENDATIONS

SETTING	SATISFACTORY	UNSATISFACTORY	SPECIFY DEFICIENCIES
LABORATORY	☐ Can now perform skill under direct clinical supervision	☐ Requires additional laboratory practice	
CLINIC	☐ Ready for minimally supervised application and refinement	☐ Requires additional supervised clinical practice ☐ Complete re-evaluation required ☐ Re-evaluation·minor deficiencies only	

STUDENT: EVALUATOR: FACULTY:

PROCEDURAL SPECIFICATIONS
MEDICAL RECORDS

I. Key Performance Elements

Unlike the observational orientation emphasized for other procedures described in this Manual, your application and evaluation
of a patient's medical record is assessed mainly by oral interaction with your evaluator. The steps described in the accompanying Proficiency Evaluation Form require that you demonstrate your ability to locate and describe the key elements of the
history, management, and progress of a patient receiving respiratory care. You will further be expected to apply this
knowledge in the development of a care plan specific to the
needs of the patient in question. For this reason, evaluation of
your proficiency in the use of the medical record is almost
entirely outcome oriented. Detailed specifications on these
expected outcomes are provided below.

II. Setting

The student is expected to demonstrate proficiency in the use
and application of medical records in the following settings:
(check those that apply)

☐ Laboratory   ☐ Other (specify)

☐ Clinic

_____

_____

III. Conditions

The student is expected to demonstrate proficiency in the use
and application of medical records under the following conditions:
(check those that apply)

Patient Variables	Type of Care
☐ Infant	☐ General therapeutics
☐ Child	☐ Critical/Intensive care
☐ Adult	☐ Rehabilitation/Long-term care

Other conditional specifications: _____

_____

_____

IV. Equipment

Not applicable

V. Outcome Criteria

Outcome criteria applicable to the use of the medical record include: (1) accuracy, (2) comprehension, and (3) application.

Accuracy of medical record utilization requires that the student make chart entries in accordance with the policies and procedures of the applicable institution and department.

Comprehension of the key elements of the patient's medical record requires the student to locate, identify, and correctly summarize the information deemed pertinent to the respiratory care of the patient.

Application of medical record information requires the student to evaluate the patient's problem(s), assess current therapies, and organize a tentative respiratory care plan which includes specification of both therapeutic alternatives and desired outcome(s) of treatment.

VI. Oral Review Questions

1. What is the policy of the institution or department regarding the following practices?
   a. student entries/signatures
   b. entries made on the wrong chart
   c. erasure of errors
   d. blank lines on continuous "notes"
   e. use of abbreviations
   f. notification of others
   g. use of ditto marks
   h. use of colored ink

2. What legal and ethical considerations must be taken into account when one is responsible for a patient's medical record?

3. How does problem-oriented medical record keeping differ from the more traditional approaches to documenting patient management?

INFECTION CONTROL

STUDENT:	DATE:				

| PROCEDURE (TASK): HANDWASHING |

SETTING: ☐ LABORATORY ☐ OTHER: (SPECIFY) ☐ CLINIC	SATISFACTORY	UNSATISFACTORY	NOT OBSERVED	NOT APPLICABLE
CONDITIONS (DESCRIBE)				
EQUIPMENT UTILIZED:				

STEPS IN PROCEDURE OR TASK:

	SATISFACTORY	UNSATISFACTORY	NOT OBSERVED	NOT APPLICABLE
PREPARATION	▨	▨	▨	▨
1. Removes jewelry				
2. Prevents clothing contact with sink				
3. Turns water on (warm)				
IMPLEMENTATION	▨	▨	▨	▨
4. Wets hands				
5. Applies soap/disinfectant thoroughly				
6. Washes palms/back of hands with rotary motion (20 sec.)				
7. Washes fingers/spaces with interlacing motion (10 sec.)				
8. Washes wrists and above (4 in.) with rotary motion				
9. Repeats steps 5 through 8				
10. Rinses well from wrists to fingers				
11. Dries with aseptic towel				
FOLLOW-UP	▨	▨	▨	▨
12. Turns off water aseptically				
13. Discards materials in receptacle				
14. Repeats procedure if contaminated				

STUDENT'S COMPREHENSION OF PROCEDURE (SELECT ONE ONLY)

The student demonstrates comprehensive knowledge of basic and advanced concepts beyond requirements of procedure	
The student demonstrates above average understanding of basic concepts applicable to the skill demonstrated	
The student demonstrates adequate knowledge of the essential elements of the task performed	
The student shows limited understanding of essential concepts related to the procedure	
The student has inadequate knowledge of even the basic concepts related to the task at hand	

OUTCOME CRITERIA (WHERE APPLICABLE)

☐ MET	SPECIFY CRITERIA NOT MET AND/OR PERTINENT CONSTRAINTS
☐ NOT MET	
☐ NOT APPL.	

ADDITIONAL COMMENTS

Include errors of omission or commission; if clinical therapeutic procedure emphasize communicative skills (verbal and non-verbal) and effectiveness of patient interaction:

SUMMARY PERFORMANCE EVALUATION AND RECOMMENDATIONS

SETTING	SATISFACTORY	UNSATISFACTORY	SPECIFY DEFICIENCIES
LABORATORY	☐ Can now perform skill under direct clinical supervision	☐ Requires additional laboratory practice	
CLINIC	☐ Ready for minimally supervised application and refinement	☐ Requires additional supervised clinical practice ☐ Complete re-evaluation required ☐ Re-evaluation·minor deficiencies only	

STUDENT: EVALUATOR: FACULTY:

PROCEDURAL SPECIFICATIONS
HANDWASHING

I. Key Performance Elements .

Procedural Element (Step)	Description of Satisfactory Performance
5. Applies soap/disinfectant thoroughly	Selects bacteriocidal scrub solution Applies solution under nails, between fingers
9. Repeats steps 5 through 8	Scrubs for 2 minutes for isolation procedures, equipment assembly Uses short scrub for routine procedures only

II. Setting

The student is expected to demonstrate proficiency in hand-washing technique in the following settings: (check those that apply)

☐ Laboratory   ☐ Other (specify)

☐ Clinic   _____

                      _____

III. Conditions

The student is expected to demonstrate proficiency in hand-washing technique under the following conditions: (check those that apply)

Procedural Variables

☐ Routine therapeutics   ☐ Aseptic equipment assembly

☐ Isolation   ☐ Strict surgical asepsis

Other conditional specifications: _____

_____

_____

IV. Equipment

The student is expected to demonstrate proficiency in hand-washing technique using the following equipment: (check those that apply)

☐ Standard sink

☐ Surgical scrub sink

☐ Disinfectant dispenser

☐ Other (specify): _____

_____

V. Outcome Criteria

Where regularly performed, bacterial cultures taken from the hands of the student should be negative for pathogens.

VI. Oral Review Questions

1. What is the rationale for handwashing between patient procedures?

2. Explain the cycle of contamination that can occur with either inanimate or animate vectors.

3. What is a nosocomial infection, and how can the occurrence of such infections be minimized by respiratory therapy personnel?

STUDENT:		DATE:			

PROCEDURE (TASK): CHEMICAL DISINFECTION AND STERILIZATION

SETTING: ☐ LABORATORY ☐ OTHER: (SPECIFY) ☐ CLINIC	SATISFACTORY	UNSATISFACTORY	NOT OBSERVED	NOT APPLICABLE
CONDITIONS (DESCRIBE)				
EQUIPMENT UTILIZED:				

STEPS IN PROCEDURE OR TASK:				
EQUIPMENT PROCUREMENT AND PREPARATION				
1. Isolates, gathers and transports equipment to site				
2. Disinfects sinks (washer)				
3. Fills wash sink, adds detergent				
4. Sorts, disassembles equipment				
5. Immerses and scrubs equipment (institutes wash cycle)				
6. Rinses equipment (institutes rinse cycle)				
7. Drains equipment				
DISINFECTION/STERILIZATION				
8. Checks solution expiration date				
9. Immerses equipment in solution (institutes disinfection cycle)				
10. Soaks equipment for specified interval				
11. Drains and rinses equipment (institutes rinse cycle)				
12. Dries equipment (institutes spin dry cycle)				
FOLLOW-UP				
13. Washes hands				
14. Reassembles equipment				
15. Cultures equipment sample(s)				
16. Bags, seals, labels, dates equipment				
17. Stores equipment, rotates stock				

STUDENT'S COMPREHENSION OF PROCEDURE (SELECT ONE ONLY)

The student demonstrates comprehensive knowledge of basic and advanced concepts beyond requirements of procedure	
The student demonstrates above average understanding of basic concepts applicable to the skill demonstrated	
The student demonstrates adequate knowledge of the essential elements of the task performed	
The student shows limited understanding of essential concepts related to the procedure	
The student has inadequate knowledge of even the basic concepts related to the task at hand	

OUTCOME CRITERIA (WHERE APPLICABLE)

☐ MET	SPECIFY CRITERIA NOT MET AND/OR PERTINENT CONSTRAINTS
☐ NOT MET	
☐ NOT APPL.	

ADDITIONAL COMMENTS

Include errors of omission or commission; if clinical therapeutic procedure emphasize communicative skills (verbal and non-verbal) and effectiveness of patient interaction:

SUMMARY PERFORMANCE EVALUATION AND RECOMMENDATIONS

SETTING	SATISFACTORY	UNSATISFACTORY	SPECIFY DEFICIENCIES
LABORATORY	☐ Can now perform skill under direct clinical super-vision	☐ Requires additional laboratory practice	
CLINIC	☐ Ready for min-imally supervised application and refinement	☐ Requires additional supervised clinical practice ☐ Complete re-evaluation required ☐ Re-evaluation·minor deficiencies only	

STUDENT: EVALUATOR: FACULTY:

PROCEDURAL SPECIFICATIONS
CHEMICAL DISINFECTION AND STERILIZATION

I. Key Performance Elements

Procedural Element (Step)	Description of Satisfactory Performance
1. Isolates, gathers, and transports equipment to site	Empties fluid reservoirs of equipment Places equipment in plastic bags Double bags equipment from isolation areas, sterilizes immediately Seals bag Avoids clean areas
2. Disinfects sinks (washer)	Selects surface disinfectant Applies disinfectant with clean towel/sponge
3. Fills wash sink, adds detergent	Uses hot water Selects detergent/disinfectant solution or powder Adds proper concentration of detergent/disinfectant
4. Sorts, disassembles equipment	Discards disposable equipment Separates out nonimmersible equipment Surface disinfects nonimmersible equipment Disassembles equipment into smallest components
5. Immerses and scrubs equipment (institutes wash cycle)	Agitates equipment to ensure exposure Removes all debris
6. Rinses equipment (institutes rinse cycle)	Uses hot water Provides double rinse Removes detergent/disinfectant residue

8. Check solution expiration date — Replaces (activates) solution if expired

9. Immerses equipment in solution (institutes disinfection cycle) — Prevents bubbles, air pockets
Exposes all surfaces to solution

10. Soaks equipment for specified time interval — Follows solution manufacturer's specifications for disinfection or sterilization

11. Drains and rinses equipment (institutes rinse cycle) — Minimizes loss of solution
Uses hot water rinse
Removes all solution residue

12. Dries equipment (institutes spin dry cycle) — Uses disinfected surface(s)
Provides for filtered airflow
Takes precautions for heat-labile equipment

13. Washes hands — Refer to proficiency evaluation: HANDWASHING (full 2 minute scrub)

14. Reassembles equipment — Maintains asepsis
Recycles contaminated equipment

15. Cultures equipment sample(s) — Refer to proficiency evaluation: BACTERIOLOGICAL SURVEILLANCE

II. Setting

The student is expected to demonstrate proficiency in the chemical disinfection and/or sterilization of equipment in the following settings: (check those that apply)

☐ Laboratory   ☐ Other (specify)

☐ Clinic

_____

_____

III. Conditions

The student is expected to demonstrate proficiency in the chemical disinfection and/or sterilization of equipment under the following conditions: (check those that apply)

Equipment Source Variables | Procedure Variables

☐ Standard (nonsuspect) recycling

☐ Disinfection only

☐ Isolation sources

☐ Sterilization

Other conditional specifications: _____

_____

_____

IV. Equipment

The student is expected to demonstrate proficiency in the chemical disinfection and/or sterilization of equipment with the following equipment: (check those that apply)

☐ Disinfectant immersion tub(s)

☐ Automated disinfectant system

☐ Forced air drying cabinet

☐ Laminar flow hood

V. Outcome Criteria

All processed equipment must be properly bagged, sealed, labeled, dated, and stored according to departmental protocol. Where performed, bacterial cultures taken from processes equipment must be negative for growth.

VI. Oral Review Questions

1. What is the difference between disinfection and sterilization?

2. What are the chemical characteristics and mode of action of the disinfection/sterilizing solution used?

3. Against which microorganisms, and under which conditions, is the solution used effective as a disinfectant? as a sterilizing agent?

4. What are the hazards involved in using the specified solution?

5. What are the advantages and limitations of chemical disinfection and/or sterilization?

STUDENT:		DATE:

PROCEDURE (TASK): GAS STERILIZATION

SETTING: ☐ LABORATORY ☐ OTHER: (SPECIFY) ☐ CLINIC	SATISFACTORY	UNSATISFACTORY	NOT OBSERVED	NOT APPLICABLE
CONDITIONS (DESCRIBE)				
EQUIPMENT UTILIZED:				

STEPS IN PROCEDURE OR TASK:				
EQUIPMENT PROCUREMENT AND PREPARATION				
1. Isolates, gathers, and transports equipment to site				
2. Disinfects sinks (washer)				
3. Fills wash sink, adds detergent				
4. Sorts, disassembles equipment				
5. Immerses and scrubs equipment (institutes wash cycle)				
6. Rinses equipment (institutes rinse cycle)				
7. Dries equipment				
8. Washes hands				
9. Reassembles equipment				
10. Bags, seals, labels, dates equipment				
STERILIZATION				
11. Inserts equipment in sterilizer with indicator				
12. Runs and logs sterilization cycle				
FOLLOW-UP				
13. Aerates equipment				
14. Incubates test indicator				
15. Verifies sterility				
16. Stores equipment, rotates stock				

STUDENT'S COMPREHENSION OF PROCEDURE (SELECT ONE ONLY)

The student demonstrates comprehensive knowledge of basic and advanced concepts beyond requirements of procedure	
The student demonstrates above average understanding of basic concepts applicable to the skill demonstrated	
The student demonstrates adequate knowledge of the essential elements of the task performed	
The student shows limited understanding of essential concepts related to the procedure	
The student has inadequate knowledge of even the basic concepts related to the task at hand	

OUTCOME CRITERIA (WHERE APPLICABLE)

☐ MET	SPECIFY CRITERIA NOT MET AND/OR PERTINENT CONSTRAINTS
☐ NOT MET	
☐ NOT APPL.	

ADDITIONAL COMMENTS

Include errors of omission or commission; if clinical therapeutic procedure emphasize communicative skills (verbal and non-verbal) and effectiveness of patient interaction:

SUMMARY PERFORMANCE EVALUATION AND RECOMMENDATIONS

SETTING	SATISFACTORY	UNSATISFACTORY	SPECIFY DEFICIENCIES
LABORATORY	☐ Can now perform skill under direct clinical supervision	☐ Requires additional laboratory practice	

CLINIC	☐ Ready for minimally supervised application and refinement	☐ Requires additional supervised clinical practice
		  ☐ Complete re-evaluation required
		  ☐ Re-evaluation·minor deficiencies only	

STUDENT: EVALUATOR: FACULTY:

PROCEDURAL SPECIFICATIONS
GAS STERILIZATION

I. Key Performance Elements

Procedural Element (Step)	Description of Satisfactory Performance
1. Isolates, gathers, and transports equipment to site	Empties fluid reservoirs of equipment Places equipment in plastic bags Double bags equipment from isolation areas, sterilizes immediately Seals bags Avoids clean areas
2. Disinfects sinks (washer)	Selects surface disinfectant Applies disinfectant with clean towel/sponge
3. Fills wash sink, adds detergent	Uses hot water Selects detergent/disinfectant solution or powder Adds proper concentration of detergent/disinfectant
4. Sorts, disassembles equipment	Discards disposable equipment Separates out nonimmersible equipment Disassembles equipment into smallest components
5. Immerses and scrubs equip- (institute wash cycle)	Agitates equipment to ensure exposure Removes all debris
6. Rinses equipment (institutes rinse cycle)	Uses hot water Provides double rinse Removes detergent/disinfectant residue
8. Washes hands	Refer to proficiency evaluation: HANDWASHING (full 2 minute scrub)

9. Reassembles equipment

Uses disinfected surface(s)
Uses laminar flow hood (where
applicable)

10. Bags, seals, labels, dates
equipment

Uses polyethylene wrap
Evacuates excess air from
bags
Ensures proper bag seal
Attaches indicator tap
Labels each bag with cycle,
cycle date, expiration
date

11. Inserts equipment in sterili-
zer with indicator

Fills chamber without
cramping
Selects unexpired bio-
logical indicator
Label indicator with cycle,
cycle date

12. Runs and logs sterilization cycle

Ensures proper humidification
Selects proper time interval
and temperature
Activates gas cartridge
Rechecks chamber seal
Logs cycle

13. Aerates equipment

Ensures gas evacuation
Sorts out metal, glass parts
requiring no aeration
Selects proper aeration time,
temperature
Ensures sufficient aeration
time

16. Stores equipment, rotates
stock

Rechecks integrity of packaging
Recycles expired stock

II. Setting

The student is expected to demonstrate proficiency in the gas
sterilization of equipment in the following settings: (check those
that apply)

☐ Laboratory

☐ Clinic

☐ Other (specify)

_____

_____

III. Conditions

The student is expected to demonstrate proficiency in the gas sterilization of equipment under the following conditions: (check those that apply)

Equipment Source Variables   Procedure Variables

☐ Standard (nonsuspect)   ☐ Ambient aeration
  recycling
☐ Isolation sources   ☐ Forced air aeration

Other conditional specifications: _____

_____

_____

IV. Equipment

The student is expected to demonstrate proficiency in the gas sterilization of equipment with the following equipment: (check those that apply)

☐ Automated sterilization chamber

☐ Forced air aeration chamber

☐ Heat sealing packaging system

☐ Other (specify): _____

_____

V. Outcome Criteria

All processed equipment must be properly bagged, sealed, labeled, dated, and stored according to departmental protocol. After completion of the processing cycle (and appropriate incubation period) the biological test indicator must be negative for growth and sample cultures taken from processed equipment must be sterile.

VI. Oral Review Questions

1. Describe the method of action and key variables affecting the efficacy of ethylene oxide sterilization.

2. What are the major hazards of ethylene oxide sterilization and how can they be minimized?

3. What are the advantages and disadvantages of ethylene oxide sterilization in comparison to other methods of disinfection/ sterilization?

4. What problems may be encountered using ethylene oxide with:
   a. inadequately dried equipment?
   b. packaging material other than polyethylene?
   c. equipment previously gamma irradiated?

STUDENT:	DATE:

PROCEDURE (TASK): PASTEURIZATION

SETTING: ☐ LABORATORY ☐ OTHER: (SPECIFY) ☐ CLINIC	SATISFACTORY	UNSATISFACTORY	NOT OBSERVED	NOT APPLICABLE
CONDITIONS (DESCRIBE)				
EQUIPMENT UTILIZED:				

STEPS IN PROCEDURE OR TASK:

	SATISFACTORY	UNSATISFACTORY	NOT OBSERVED	NOT APPLICABLE
EQUIPMENT PROCUREMENT AND PREPARATION	▨	▨	▨	▨
1. Isolates, gathers, and transports equipment to site				
2. Disinfects sink (washer)				
3. Fills wash sink, adds detergent				
4. Sorts, disassembles equipment				
5. Immerses and scrubs equipment (institutes wash cycle)				
6. Rinses equipment (institutes rinse cycle)				
7. Drains equipment				
PASTEURIZATION	▨	▨	▨	▨
8. Confirms water bath temperature				
9. Immerses equipment in water bath				
10. Soaks equipment for specified interval				
11. Drains equipment				
12. Dries equipment				
FOLLOW-UP	▨	▨	▨	▨
13. Washes hands				
14. Reassembles equipment				
15. Cultures equipment sample(s)				
16. Bags, seals, labels, dates equipment				
17. Stores equipment, rotates stock				

STUDENT'S COMPREHENSION OF PROCEDURE (SELECT ONE ONLY)

The student demonstrates comprehensive knowledge of basic and advanced concepts beyond requirements of procedure	
The student demonstrates above average understanding of basic concepts applicable to the skill demonstrated	
The student demonstrates adequate knowledge of the essential elements of the task performed	
The student shows limited understanding of essential concepts related to the procedure	
The student has inadequate knowledge of even the basic concepts related to the task at hand	

OUTCOME CRITERIA (WHERE APPLICABLE)

☐ MET	SPECIFY CRITERIA NOT MET AND/OR PERTINENT CONSTRAINTS
☐ NOT MET	
☐ NOT APPL.	

ADDITIONAL COMMENTS

Include errors of omission or commission; if clinical therapeutic procedure emphasize communicative skills (verbal and non-verbal) and effectiveness of patient interaction:

SUMMARY PERFORMANCE EVALUATION AND RECOMMENDATIONS

SETTING	SATISFACTORY	UNSATISFACTORY	SPECIFY DEFICIENCIES
LABORATORY	☐ Can now perform skill under direct clinical super-vision	☐ Requires additional laboratory practice	
CLINIC	☐ Ready for min-imally supervised application and refinement	☐ Requires additional supervised clinical practice 　☐ Complete re-evaluation required 　☐ Re-evaluation·minor deficiencies only	

STUDENT:　　　　　EVALUATOR:　　　　FACULTY:

PROCEDURAL SPECIFICATIONS
PASTEURIZATION

I. Key Performance Elements

Procedural Element (Step)	Description of Satisfactory Performance
1. Isolates, gathers, and transports equipment to site	Empties fluid reservoirs of equipment Places equipment in plastic bags Double bags equipment from isolation areas, sterilizes immediately Seals bags Avoids clean areas
2. Disinfects sinks (washer)	Selects surface disinfectant Applies disinfectant with clean towel/sponge
3. Fills wash sink, adds detergent	Uses hot water Selects detergent/disinfectant solution or powder Adds proper concentration of detergent/disinfectant
4. Sorts, disassembles equipment	Discards disposable equipment Separates out nonimmersible equipment Surface disinfects nonimmersible equipment Disassembles equipment into smallest components
5. Immerses and scrubs equipment (institutes wash cycle)	Agitates equipment to ensure exposure Removes all debris
6. Rinses equipment (institutes rinse cycle)	Uses hot water Provides double rinse Removes detergent/disinfectant residue
8. Confirms water bath temperature	Ensures 170° F

9. Immerses equipment in water bath

Prevents bubbles, air pockets
Exposes all surfaces to water

10. Soaks equipment for specified interval

Adheres to 30 minute minimum or specification of manufacturer

12. Dries equipment

Uses disinfected surface(s)
Provides for filtered airflow
Takes precautions for heat-labile equipment

13. Washes hands

Refer to proficiency evaluation: HANDWASHING

14. Reassembles equipment

Maintains asepsis
Recycles contaminated equipment

15. Cultures equipment sample(s)

Refer to proficiency evaluation: BACTERIOLOGICAL SURVEILLANCE

II. Setting

The student is expected to demonstrate proficiency in the pasteurization of equipment in the following settings: (check those that apply)

☐ Laboratory

☐ Other (specify)

☐ Clinic

_____

_____

III. Conditions

The student is expected to demonstrate proficiency in the pasteurization of equipment under the following conditions: (check those that apply)

Equipment Source Variables

☐ Standard (nonsuspect) recycling

☐ Isolation sources

Other conditional specifications: _____

_____

_____

IV. Equipment

The student is expected to demonstrate proficiency in the pasteurization of equipment using the following equipment: (check those that apply)

☐ Manually operated water bath

☐ Automated pasteurization system

☐ Forced air drying cabinet

☐ Laminar flow hood

V. Outcome Criteria

All processed equipment must be properly bagged, sealed, labeled, dated, and stored according to departmental protocol. Where performed, bacterial cultures taken from processed equipment must be negative for common respiratory pathogens.

VI. Oral Review Questions

1. Describe the method of action and key variables affecting the efficacy of pasteurization.

2. Against which microorganisms is pasteurization not effective as a disinfection process?

3. What are the advantages and limitations of pasteurization over other methods of disinfection and sterilization?

4. When is recontamination of equipment during the pasteurization process most likely to occur? How can the likelihood of recontamination be minimized?

STUDENT:	DATE:				

PROCEDURE (TASK): BACTERIOLOGICAL SURVEILLANCE					

	SATISFACTORY	UNSATISFACTORY	NOT OBSERVED	NOT APPLICABLE
SETTING: ☐ LABORATORY ☐ OTHER: (SPECIFY) ☐ CLINIC				
CONDITIONS (DESCRIBE)				
EQUIPMENT UTILIZED:				
STEPS IN PROCEDURE OR TASK:				
EQUIPMENT PREPARATION				
1. Selects and gathers appropriate equipment				
2. Checks (ensures) sterility of sampling and transfer apparatus				
3. Washes hands				
4. Opens sampling (culture transfer) packaging				
SAMPLING PROCEDURE				
5. Selects appropriate location/technique for obtaining sample				
6. Obtain adequate sample aseptically				
7. Labels, logs sample as to equipment, location, status, date				
8. Isolates sample				
9. Transfers sample to culture/growth media				
10. Incubates sample (delivers to laboratory)				
FOLLOW-UP				
11. Monitors culture media for bacteriological growth (secures lab report				
12. Evaluates presence/nature of bacteriological growth (lab report)				
13. Takes appropriate action				
14. Maintains records/results of actions taken				

STUDENT'S COMPREHENSION OF PROCEDURE (SELECT ONE ONLY)

The student demonstrates comprehensive knowledge of basic and advanced concepts beyond requirements of procedure	
The student demonstrates above average understanding of basic concepts applicable to the skill demonstrated	
The student demonstrates adequate knowledge of the essential elements of the task performed	
The student shows limited understanding of essential concepts related to the procedure	
The student has inadequate knowledge of even the basic concepts related to the task at hand	

OUTCOME CRITERIA (WHERE APPLICABLE)

☐ MET	SPECIFY CRITERIA NOT MET AND/OR PERTINENT CONSTRAINTS
☐ NOT MET	
☐ NOT APPL.	

ADDITIONAL COMMENTS

Include errors of omission or commission; if clinical therapeutic procedure emphasize communicative skills (verbal and non-verbal) and effectiveness of patient interaction:

SUMMARY PERFORMANCE EVALUATION AND RECOMMENDATIONS

SETTING	SATISFACTORY	UNSATISFACTORY	SPECIFY DEFICIENCIES
LABORATORY	☐ Can now perform skill under direct clinical supervision	☐ Requires additional laboratory practice	
CLINIC	☐ Ready for minimally supervised application and refinement	☐ Requires additional supervised clinical practice ☐ Complete re-evaluation required ☐ Re-evaluation·minor deficiencies only	

STUDENT: EVALUATOR: FACULTY:

PROCEDURAL SPECIFICATIONS
BACTERIOLOGICAL SURVEILLANCE

I. Key Performance Elements

Procedural Element (Step)	Description of Satisfactory Performance
1. Selects and gathers appropriate equipment	Chooses sampling/transfer apparatus appropriate to task at hand, i.e., swabs/plates for surface sampling; aliquot tubes for reservoir sampling; impaction collectors for effluent aerosol sampling
2. Checks (ensures) sterility of sampling and transfer apparatus	Confirms packaging seal/sterility label Checks expiration date
3. Washes hands	Refer to proficiency evaluation: HANDWASHING
4. Opens sampling (culture transfer) packaging	Prevents contact/contamination
5. Selects appropriate location/technique for obtaining sample	Swabs or contact plates surfaces Remove aliquot from liquid reservoirs Collects effluent aerosol by impaction
13. Takes appropriate action	Informs epidemiologist of culture results Identifies potential sources of contamination (if present) Eliminates contamination sources Rechecks/verifies cleaning/disinfection/sterilization processes

II. Setting

The student is expected to demonstrate proficiency in the application of bacteriological surveillance procedures in the following settings: (check those that apply)

☐ Laboratory   ☐ Other (specify)

☐ Clinic

_____

_____

III. Conditions

The student is expected to demonstrate proficiency in the application of bacteriological surveillance procedures under the following conditions: (check those that apply)

Sampling Variables   Procedure Variables

☐ Surface samples   ☐ Departmental culturing

☐ Fluid reservoir samples   ☐ Laboratory culturing

☐ Effluent gas (aerosol) samples

Other conditional specifications: _____

_____

_____

IV. Equipment

The student is expected to demonstrate proficiency in the application of bacteriological surveillance procedures using the following equipment: (check those that apply)

☐ Swab sampling kit

☐ Surface plate sampling kit

☐ Aerosol impaction collector system

☐ Incubator

☐ Other (specify): _____

_____

V. Outcome Criteria

Given a positive sample result and appropriate documentation (sterilization logs, equipment usage, infection reports, etc.), the student will identify the potential sources of contamination and recommend means of eliminating such sources.

VI. Oral Review Questions

1. What is the rationale for bacteriological surveillance of respiratory therapy equipment?

2. What are the organisms most frequently contaminating respiratory therapy equipment? What environmental factors enhance their growth?

3. What patient categories are most susceptible to nosocomial infection?

4. What are the key elements in a systematic plan to minimize nosocomial infections in a hospital?

STUDENT:		DATE:				

PROCEDURE (TASK): ISOLATION					

SETTING: ☐ LABORATORY ☐ OTHER: (SPECIFY) ☐ CLINIC	SATISFACTORY	UNSATISFACTORY	NOT OBSERVED	NOT APPLICABLE
CONDITIONS (DESCRIBE)				
EQUIPMENT UTILIZED:				

STEPS IN PROCEDURE OR TASK:	SATISFACTORY	UNSATISFACTORY	NOT OBSERVED	NOT APPLICABLE
PREPARATION	▨	▨	▨	▨
1. Verifies type, nature and purpose of isolation				
2. Washes hands				
3. Selects and gathers appropriate equipment				
IMPLEMENTATION	▨	▨	▨	▨
4. Dons protective shoe/hair coverings				
5. Dons, closes, and fastens gown				
6. Applies mask				
7. Dons gloves over gown				
8. Enters room, explains procedure to patient				
9. Performs duties, reassures patient				
10. Discards contaminated supplies				
11. Bags, seals, labels, and transfers contaminated equipment				
12. Removes, discards shoe coverings, gloves				
13. Unfastens gown				
14. Removes, discards gown, mask, haircovering				
FOLLOW-UP	▨	▨	▨	▨
15. Washes hands				
16. Maintains/processes equipment				
17. Records pertinent data in chart and departmental records				
18. Notifies appropriate personnel				

STUDENT'S COMPREHENSION OF PROCEDURE (SELECT ONE ONLY)

The student demonstrates comprehensive knowledge of basic and advanced concepts beyond requirements of procedure	
The student demonstrates above average understanding of basic concepts applicable to the skill demonstrated	
The student demonstrates adequate knowledge of the essential elements of the task performed	
The student shows limited understanding of essential concepts related to the procedure	
The student has inadequate knowledge of even the basic concepts related to the task at hand	

OUTCOME CRITERIA (WHERE APPLICABLE)

☐ MET	SPECIFY CRITERIA NOT MET AND/OR PERTINENT CONSTRAINTS
☐ NOT MET	
☐ NOT APPL.	

ADDITIONAL COMMENTS

Include errors of omission or commission; if clinical therapeutic procedure emphasize communicative skills (verbal and non-verbal) and effectiveness of patient interaction:

SUMMARY PERFORMANCE EVALUATION AND RECOMMENDATIONS

SETTING	SATISFACTORY	UNSATISFACTORY	SPECIFY DEFICIENCIES
LABORATORY	☐ Can now perform skill under direct clinical super-vision	☐ Requires additional laboratory practice	
CLINIC	☐ Ready for min-imally supervised application and refinement	☐ Requires additional supervised clinical practice ☐ Complete re-evaluation required ☐ Re-evaluation·minor deficiencies only	

STUDENT: EVALUATOR: FACULTY:

PROCEDURAL SPECIFICATIONS
ISOLATION

I. Key Performance Elements

Procedural Element (Step)	Description of Satisfactory Performance
2. Washes hands	Refer to proficiency evaluation: HANDWASHING
5. Dons, closes, and fastens gown	Holds gown at neck opening, unfolds downward Puts arms through gown sleeves, touching inside only Adjusts gown on shoulders, working from inside only Ties neck tapes without touching hair Draws rear edges, ties waist belt
7. Dons gloves over gown	Unfolds glove wrapper without touching gloves Grasps inside folded edge of cufftop with dominant hand Pulls glove over opposite hand, touching inside only Grasps outside folded edge of cufftop with gloved hand Pulls glove over dominant hand, touching inside only Adjusts fingers of gloves
11. Bags, seal, labels, and transfers contaminated equipment	Uses double-bag method Transfers bagged equipment out of room Labels as contaminated
12. Removes, discards shoe coverings, gloves	Prevents mask contact with gown Removes right-hand glove by cuff with left hand without touching skin Pulls left-hand glove off with fingers of right hand inside glove cuff Discards gloves/mask in designated container

14. Removes, discards gown,
mask, haircovering

Works gown off with hands
under cuffs of sleeves
Discards gown in soiled linen
hamper in patient's room
Avoids contamination

II. Setting

The student is expected to demonstrate proficiency in the application of isolation procedures in the following settings: (check those that apply)

☐ Laboratory

☐ Clinic

☐ Other (specify)

_____

_____

III. Conditions

The student is expected to demonstrate proficiency in the application of isolation procedures under the following conditions: (check those that apply)

Isolation Type Variables	Procedure Variables
☐ Standard	☐ Equipment change or gathering only
☐ Reverse	☐ Low risk procedures (i.e., oxygen therapy, etc.)
☐ Enteric	☐ High risk procedures (i.e., airway care, arterial sampling, etc.)
☐ Wound/skin	
☐ Respiratory	

Other conditional specifications: _____

_____

_____

IV. Equipment

Not applicable

V. Outcome Criteria

All disposable equipment and protective wear is discarded in the appropriate receptacle(s). All contaminated nondisposable equipment is double bagged, labeled, and processed according to departmental protocol.

VI. Oral Review Questions

1. Specify the requirements (room, gowns, masks, hands, gloves, and special precautions governing articles of use) and identify 3–4 medical or surgical conditions associated with each of the following categories of isolation:
   a. standard (complete) isolation
   b. reverse (protective) isolation
   c. enteric isolation
   d. wound/skin isolation
   e. respiratory isolation

MEDICAL GAS THERAPY

STUDENT:	DATE:				

PROCEDURE (TASK): CYLINDER SAFETY AND TRANSPORT

	SATISFACTORY	UNSATISFACTORY	NOT OBSERVED	NOT APPLICABLE
SETTING: ☐ LABORATORY ☐ OTHER: (SPECIFY) ☐ CLINIC				
CONDITIONS (DESCRIBE)				
EQUIPMENT UTILIZED:				

STEPS IN PROCEDURE OR TASK:	SATISFACTORY	UNSATISFACTORY	NOT OBSERVED	NOT APPLICABLE
EQUIPMENT PREPARATION	▨	▨	▨	▨
1. Selects appropriate cylinder (size, content)				
2. Maneuvers cylinder properly to cart or stand				
3. Secures cylinder				
4. Removes valve stem cap or cover				
5. Cracks cylinder				
IMPLEMENTATION	▨	▨	▨	▨
6. Selects appropriate regulator				
7. Attaches regulator to cylinder valve stem				
8. Slowly opens cylinder valve				
9. Checks regulator/cylinder assembly for leakage/fit				
10. Reads cylinder contents				
11. Estimates duration of flow for specified use				
12. Transports cylinder properly to destination				
13. Connects specified equipment to regulator				
14. Follows oxygen safety precautions (where applicable)				
FOLLOW-UP	▨	▨	▨	▨
15. Schedules cylinder content check/change at correct time				
16. If gas not in use, turns cylinder valve off, evacuates regulator				

STUDENT'S COMPREHENSION OF PROCEDURE (SELECT ONE ONLY)

The student demonstrates comprehensive knowledge of basic and advanced concepts beyond requirements of procedure	
The student demonstrates above average understanding of basic concepts applicable to the skill demonstrated	
The student demonstrates adequate knowledge of the essential elements of the task performed	
The student shows limited understanding of essential concepts related to the procedure	
The student has inadequate knowledge of even the basic concepts related to the task at hand	

OUTCOME CRITERIA (WHERE APPLICABLE)

☐ MET	SPECIFY CRITERIA NOT MET AND/OR PERTINENT CONSTRAINTS
☐ NOT MET	
☐ NOT APPL.	

ADDITIONAL COMMENTS

Include errors of omission or commission; if clinical therapeutic procedure emphasize communicative skills (verbal and non-verbal) and effectiveness of patient interaction:

SUMMARY PERFORMANCE EVALUATION AND RECOMMENDATIONS

SETTING	SATISFACTORY	UNSATISFACTORY	SPECIFY DEFICIENCIES
LABORATORY	☐ Can now perform skill under direct clinical super-vision	☐ Requires additional laboratory practice	

CLINIC	☐ Ready for min-imally supervised application and refinement	☐ Requires additional supervised clinical practice
		  ☐ Complete re-evaluation required
		  ☐ Re-evaluation·minor deficiencies only	

STUDENT: EVALUATOR: FACULTY:

PROCEDURAL SPECIFICATIONS
CYLINDER SAFETY AND TRANSPORT

I. Key Performance Elements

Procedural Element (Step)	Description of Satisfactory Performance
1. Select appropriate cylinder (size, content)	Identifies cylinder size appropriate to requisite duration of flow Checks cylinder color code Verifies contents with label
2. Maneuvers cylinder properly to cart or stand	Tilts cylinder approximately 15° Twists and rolls to cart, ensuring support
3. Secures cylinder	Chains cylinder to portable stand Fixes cylinder to immovable base with thumb nuts
5. Cracks cylinder	Faces valve outlet away from persons/damageable objects Twists valve quickly open, then closed
6. Selects appropriate regulator	Determines which safety systems apply to cylinder Selects regulator/metering combination appropriate to task
7. Attaches regulator to cylinder valve stem	Aligns regulator/valve stem Inserts bushing for PISS connection
12. Transports cylinder properly to destination	Supports cart with both hands Ensures cart stability in transit Proceeds cautiously

14. Follows oxygen safety precautions (where applicable)

Posts "oxygen-in-use" signs
Removes ignition sources
   from room
Informs patient and staff of
   oxygen precautions

II. Setting

The student is expected to demonstrate proficiency in the application of cylinder safety and transport procedures in the following settings: (check those that apply)

☐ Laboratory

☐ Clinic

☐ Other (specify)

_____

_____

III. Conditions

The student is expected to demonstrate proficiency in the
application of cylinder safety and transport procedures under
the following conditions: (check those that apply)

Gases

☐ Oxygen

☐ Any therapeutic gas

☐ Laboratory gases

☐ Anesthetic gases

Procedure Variables

☐ Bedside therapy

☐ Transport

☐ Manifold system

Other conditional specifications: _____

_____

_____

IV. Equipment

The student is expected to demonstrate proficiency in the application of cylinder safety and transport procedures under the following conditions: (check those that apply)

Cylinder Sizes   Regulator Types

☐ A-E (PISS)   ☐ Single stage

☐ G, H, K   ☐ Multiple stage
(American Standard)

Regulator/Metering Combinations

☐ Bourdon gauge

☐ Thorpe tube

☐ Other (specify): _____

_____

V. Outcome Criteria

The student must select the cylinder contents, size, and pressure regulating/flow metering combination appropriate to the task (as judged by the supervisor/evaluator). In addition the student's calculation of cylinder duration of flow and determination of scheduled change of cylinder must correspond to those determined by the supervisor/evaluator.

VI. Oral Review Questions

1. Who is responsible for regulating:
   a. cylinder manufacture/safety testing?
   b. medical gas purity?
   c. storage of compressed gases?

2. Identify and explain the meaning of each of the markings found on the cylinder shoulder.

3. Classify the regulator/metering system utilized in the performance of this procedure.

4. Identify the function and purpose of any/all safety systems which are part of the equipment utilized for this purpose.

5. What are the significant hazards associated with the use of compressed oxygen?

STUDENT:		DATE:			

PROCEDURE (TASK): OXYGEN THERAPY

SETTING: ☐ LABORATORY ☐ OTHER: (SPECIFY) ☐ CLINIC	SATISFACTORY	UNSATISFACTORY	NOT OBSERVED	NOT APPLICABLE
CONDITIONS (DESCRIBE)				
EQUIPMENT UTILIZED:				

STEPS IN PROCEDURE OR TASK:	SATISFACTORY	UNSATISFACTORY	NOT OBSERVED	NOT APPLICABLE
EQUIPMENT AND PATIENT PREPARATION				
1. Washes hands				
2. Selects, gathers, and assembles appropriate equipment				
3. Verifies, interprets, and evaluates physician's order				
4. Identifies patient, self, and department				
5. Explains procedure and confirms patient understanding				
IMPLEMENTATION AND ASSESSMENT				
6. Adds sterile (distilled) water to humidifier/aerosol generator				
7. Connects humidifier (aerosol generator), flowmeter, oxygen modality				
8. Initiates gas flow				
9. Tests equipment for proper function				
10. Assesses patient (objective and subjective)				
11. Applies modality to patient, ensuring maximum comfort/safety				
12. Adjusts gas flow (oxygen concentration) appropriate to orders/ objectives				
13. Assesses patient's response (objective and subjective)				
14. Modifies procedure to accommodate patient's response				
15. Analyzes F_IO_2 (where appropriate/feasible)				
16. Follows oxygen safety precautions (provides instructions to patient)				
FOLLOW-UP				
17. Maintains proper equipment function				
18. Records pertinent data in chart and department records				
19. Notifies appropriate personnel				

STUDENT'S COMPREHENSION OF PROCEDURE (SELECT ONE ONLY)

The student demonstrates comprehensive knowledge of basic and advanced concepts beyond requirements of procedure	
The student demonstrates above average understanding of basic concepts applicable to the skill demonstrated	
The student demonstrates adequate knowledge of the essential elements of the task performed	
The student shows limited understanding of essential concepts related to the procedure	
The student has inadequate knowledge of even the basic concepts related to the task at hand	

OUTCOME CRITERIA (WHERE APPLICABLE)

☐ MET	SPECIFY CRITERIA NOT MET AND/OR PERTINENT CONSTRAINTS
☐ NOT MET	
☐ NOT APPL.	

ADDITIONAL COMMENTS

Include errors of omission or commission; if clinical therapeutic procedure emphasize communicative skills (verbal and non-verbal) and effectiveness of patient interaction:

SUMMARY PERFORMANCE EVALUATION AND RECOMMENDATIONS

SETTING	SATISFACTORY	UNSATISFACTORY	SPECIFY DEFICIENCIES
LABORATORY	☐ Can now perform skill under direct clinical super-vision	☐ Requires additional laboratory practice	
CLINIC	☐ Ready for min-imally supervised application and refinement	☐ Requires additional supervised clinical practice 　☐ Complete re-evaluation required 　☐ Re-evaluation·minor deficiencies only	

STUDENT:　　　　　　　EVALUATOR:　　　　　FACULTY:

PROCEDURAL SPECIFICATIONS
OXYGEN THERAPY

I. Key Performance Elements

Procedural Element (Step)	Description of Satisfactory Performance
3. Verifies, interprets, and evaluates physician's order	Checks chart for contraindications to therapy ordered Correlates indications for oxygen with correct mode of administration
9. Tests equipment for proper functions	Checks patency of delivery system Checks operation of humidifier (aerosol generator) for proper function output Ensures operation of relief valves venturi systems, breathing valves Replaces defective or inoperable equipment/components
10. Assesses patient (objective and subjective)	Observes patient for signs/symptoms of hypoxia, to include: a. color b. breathing pattern, rate c. sensorium Measures pulse rate
11. Applies modality to patient, ensuring maximum comfort, safety	Reassures patient Applies device to airway Stabilizes device Ensures proper fit Recheck operation of valves, reservoirs
12. Adjusts gas flow (oxygen concentration) appropriate to orders/objectives	Adjust gas flow (where applicable) to ensure: a. minimal rebreathing b. sufficient reservoir volume during inspiration c. inspiratory flow demands satisfied d. desired F_IO_2 e. patient comfort

13. Assesses patient response (objective and subjective)

Observes patient for alleviation of signs/symptoms of hypoxia, to include changes in:
a. color
b. breathing pattern, rate
c. sensorium
d. pulse rate

Orders (performs) arterial blood gas

Confirms response by assessment of arterial blood gas results

14. Modifies procedure to accommodate patient's response

Increases/decreases F_IO_2 to achieve desired PaO_2

Modifies/changes mode of administration appropriate to patient's needs and therapeutic objectives

15. Analyzes F_IO_2 (where appropriate/feasible)

Refer to proficiency evaluation: MEASUREMENT OF OXYGEN CONCENTRATIONS

16. Follows oxygen safety precautions (provides instructions to patient)

Posts "oxygen-in-use" signs

Removes ignition sources from room

Informs patient and staff of oxygen precautions

II. Setting

The student is expected to demonstrate proficiency in the application of oxygen therapy in the following settings: (check those that apply)

☐ Laboratory   ☐ Other (specify)

☐ Clinic

_____

_____

III. Conditions

The student is expected to demonstrate proficiency in the application of oxygen therapy under the following conditions: (check those that apply)

Patient Variables

☐ Simulated (peer)

☐ Child

☐ Adult

Procedure Variables

☐ Humidification only

☐ In combination with aerosol

Other conditional specifications: _____

_____

IV. Equipment

The student is expected to demonstrate proficiency in the application of oxygen therapy with the following equipment: (check those that apply)

Gas Source

☐ Cylinder

☐ Bulk delivery system

☐ Other (specify)

_____

_____

Therapeutic Modality

☐ Nasal cannula

☐ Nasal catheter

☐ Simple mask

☐ Partial rebreathing mask

☐ Nonrebreathing mask

☐ Air entrainment mask

☐ T-tube (Brigg's adapter)

☐ Tracheostomy mask

V. Outcome Criteria

Where applicable, the administration of oxygen to a patient should result in achievement of the desired therapeutic objectives, e.g., alleviation of the clinical manifestations of hypoxia, a satisfactory PaO_2, etc.

VI. Oral Review Questions

1. What are the clinical indications for oxygen therapy?

2. What potentially beneficial and detrimental physiological effects can result from administration of oxygen?

3. What objective and subjective means can be used to assess achievement of the desired therapeutic outcomes of oxygen therapy? (Relate patient pathophysiology to intended goals.)

4. What possible alternatives are there to the therapy instituted? What are their advantages/disadvantages?

5. For the specific apparatus utilized, describe its functional characteristics and principles of operation.

STUDENT:	DATE:				

PROCEDURE (TASK): OXYHOOD

	SATISFACTORY	UNSATISFACTORY	NOT OBSERVED	NOT APPLICABLE
SETTING: ☐ LABORATORY ☐ OTHER: (SPECIFY) ☐ CLINIC				
CONDITIONS (DESCRIBE)				
EQUIPMENT UTILIZED:				

STEPS IN PROCEDURE OR TASK:

	SATISFACTORY	UNSATISFACTORY	NOT OBSERVED	NOT APPLICABLE
EQUIPMENT AND PATIENT PREPARATION	▨	▨	▨	▨
1. Washes hands				
2. Selects, gathers, and assembles appropriate equipment				
3. Verifies, interprets, and evaluates physician's orders				
4. Explains procedures to parents and confirms understanding				
IMPLEMENTATION AND ASSESSMENT	▨	▨	▨	▨
5. Properly fills humidifier or nebulizer with sterile, distilled water				
6. Attaches humidifier or nebulizer to appropriate gas sources				
7. Preheats humidifier/nebulizer				
8. Connects tubing to enclosure				
9. Initiates proper gas flowrate/checks for proper function				
10. Places infant in enclosure/ensures proper fit and patient comfort				
11. Analyzes F_IO_2 and ensures proper level				
12. Monitors temperature and ensures proper level				
13. Monitors and assesses patient's status/obtains objective/subjective data on oxygenation				
14. Readjust therapy as indicated				
15. Provides for continuous (if applicable) temperature and F_IO_2 monitoring				
FOLLOW-UP	▨	▨	▨	▨
16. Maintains/processes equipment				
17. Records pertinent data in chart and department records				
18. Notifies appropriate personnel				

STUDENT'S COMPREHENSION OF PROCEDURE (SELECT ONE ONLY)

The student demonstrates comprehensive knowledge of basic and advanced concepts beyond requirements of procedure	
The student demonstrates above average understanding of basic concepts applicable to the skill demonstrated	
The student demonstrates adequate knowledge of the essential elements of the task performed	
The student shows limited understanding of essential concepts related to the procedure	
The student has inadequate knowledge of even the basic concepts related to the task at hand	

OUTCOME CRITERIA (WHERE APPLICABLE)

☐ MET	SPECIFY CRITERIA NOT MET AND/OR PERTINENT CONSTRAINTS
☐ NOT MET	
☐ NOT APPL.	

ADDITIONAL COMMENTS

Include errors of omission or commission; if clinical therapeutic procedure emphasize communicative skills (verbal and non-verbal) and effectiveness of patient interaction:

SUMMARY PERFORMANCE EVALUATION AND RECOMMENDATIONS

SETTING	SATISFACTORY	UNSATISFACTORY	SPECIFY DEFICIENCIES
LABORATORY	☐ Can now perform skill under direct clinical supervision	☐ Requires additional laboratory practice	
CLINIC	☐ Ready for minimally supervised application and refinement	☐ Requires additional supervised clinical practice ☐ Complete re-evaluation required ☐ Re-evaluation·minor deficiencies only	

STUDENT: EVALUATOR: FACULTY:

PROCEDURAL SPECIFICATIONS
OXYHOOD

I. Key Performance Elements

Procedural Element (Step)	Description of Satisfactory Performance
6. Attaches humidifier or nebulizer to appropriate gas source	Selects gas source corresponding to F_IO_2 ordered If blender utilized with nebulizer, ensures that nebulizer setting is at 100% source gas
7. Preheats humidifier/nebulizer	Ensures proper function and adjustability of heating unit/checks operation of alarm indicators/safety system
8. Initiates proper gas flow-rate/checks for proper function	Sets gas flow sufficient to prevent CO_2 build up (7 LPM minimum) If nebulizer utilized, checks for sufficient aerosol production
10. Places infant in enclosure/ensures proper fit and patient comfort	Maintains patient position so that patient's head and face is away from direct gas flow Adjusts fit to provide for adequate wash-out of CO_2
11. Analyzes F_IO_2 and ensures proper level	Analyzes F_IO_2 at least once every two hours (continuously) Calibrates analyzer on 21% and 100% at least once every shift
12. Monitors temperature and ensures proper level	Provides for continuous temperature monitoring Maintains gas temperature within 1° of infant's neutral thermal environment

13. Monitors and assesses patient's status/obtains objective/subjective data on oxygenation

Ensures appropriate monitoring, to include:
Signs of respiratory distress;
a. nasal flaring
b. substernal/intercostal retractions
c. trachypnca
d. grunting
Signs of hypoxemia or cold stress;
a. vital signs
b. body temperature
c. breath sounds
d. body weight (for fluid gain)
e. arterial blood gases

II. Setting

The student is expected to demonstrate proficiency in the application of oxygen via an oxyhood in the following settings: (check those that apply)

☐ Laboratory

☐ Clinic

☐ Other (specify)

_____

_____

III. Conditions

The student is expected to demonstrate proficiency in the application of oxygen via an oxyhood under the following conditions: (check those that apply)

Patient Variables

☐ Simulated (manikin)

☐ Full term infant

☐ Preterm neonate

Procedure Variables

☐ Humidification only

☐ In combination with aerosol

Other conditional specifications: _____

_____

_____

IV. Equipment

The student is expected to demonstrate proficiency in the application of oxygen via an oxyhood using the following equipment: (check those that apply)

Enclosure Variables

☐ Simple hood

☐ Isolette

☐ Other (specify):

_____

_____

Humidification Variables

☐ Heated humidifier

☐ Heated aerosol generator

☐ Other (specify):

_____

_____

Gas Source Variables

☐ Air entrainment

☐ Blender (air and oxygen source)

Oxygen Analysis

☐ Intermittent (paramagnetic, thermal conductivity)

☐ Continuous (polaragraphic)

V. Outcome Criteria

Outcomes of oxygen administration to the infant/neonate via oxyhood should correspond, where possible, to those established by the Committee on the Fetus and Newborn of the American Academy of Pediatrics, i.e.:

If no arterial blood gas data is immediately available, oxygen should be given at concentration just high enough to abolish central cyanosis.

When arterial blood gas data is available, oxygen should be given in concentrations sufficient to maintain a PaO_2 of between 50–80 mmHg.

VI. Oral Review Questions

1. Describe the key considerations in the administration of oxygen therapy to newborn infants (as recommended by the Committee on the Fetus and Newborn of the American Academy of Pediatrics).

2. Describe the major hazards of oxygen therapy in newborn infants and children (include, where appropriate, the pathophysiology of the hazard identified).

3. Relate the problems of cold stress in newborns to oxygen administration.

4. Differentiate between the clinical indications, capabilities of, advantages, disadvantages, and limitations of the following neonatal/pediatric oxygen administration devices:
   a. oxygen hood
   b. isolette
   c. croupette/tent
   d. airway modalities (masks, etc.)

5. Identify 3–4 hazards of aerosol therapy in neonatal and pediatric patients.

STUDENT:		DATE:				

PROCEDURE (TASK): MEASUREMENT OF OXYGEN CONCENTRATIONS

	SATISFACTORY	UNSATISFACTORY	NOT OBSERVED	NOT APPLICABLE
SETTING: ☐ LABORATORY ☐ OTHER: (SPECIFY) ☐ CLINIC				
CONDITIONS (DESCRIBE)				
EQUIPMENT UTILIZED:				

STEPS IN PROCEDURE OR TASK:

	SATISFACTORY	UNSATISFACTORY	NOT OBSERVED	NOT APPLICABLE
EQUIPMENT AND PATIENT PREPARATION				
1. Selects and gathers appropriate analyzer, accessories				
2. Verifies physician's order for specified F_1O_2				
3. Identifies patient, self, department				
4. Explains procedure and confirms patient understanding				
IMPLEMENTATION				
5. Checks for proper electrical function of analyzer				
6. Check dessicant or balast (where applicable)				
7. Calibrates analyzer on room air (balance)				
8. Slopes analyzer to 100% O_2 or specific known concentration				
9. Places probe (sampling tube) in gas atmosphere				
10. Takes sample or waits for full response				
11. Makes reading				
12. Corrects for temperature, humidity or pressure (where applicable)				
13. Removes or secures probe/sampling tube				
14. Turns analyzer off				
FOLLOW-UP				
15. Records oxygen concentration in appropriate records				
16. Maintains equipment				
17. Notifies appropriate personnel				
18. Rechecks oxygen concentration as required				

STUDENT'S COMPREHENSION OF PROCEDURE (SELECT ONE ONLY)

The student demonstrates comprehensive knowledge of basic and advanced concepts beyond requirements of procedure	
The student demonstrates above average understanding of basic concepts applicable to the skill demonstrated	
The student demonstrates adequate knowledge of the essential elements of the task performed	
The student shows limited understanding of essential concepts related to the procedure	
The student has inadequate knowledge of even the basic concepts related to the task at hand	

OUTCOME CRITERIA (WHERE APPLICABLE)

☐ MET	SPECIFY CRITERIA NOT MET AND/OR PERTINENT CONSTRAINTS
☐ NOT MET	
☐ NOT APPL.	

ADDITIONAL COMMENTS

Include errors of omission or commission; if clinical therapeutic procedure emphasize communicative skills (verbal and non-verbal) and effectiveness of patient interaction:

SUMMARY PERFORMANCE EVALUATION AND RECOMMENDATIONS

SETTING	SATISFACTORY	UNSATISFACTORY	SPECIFY DEFICIENCIES
LABORATORY	☐ Can now perform skill under direct clinical super-vision	☐ Requires additional laboratory practice	
CLINIC	☐ Ready for min-imally supervised application and refinement	☐ Requires additional supervised clinical practice ☐ Complete re-evaluation required ☐ Re-evaluation·minor deficiencies only	

STUDENT:　　　　　EVALUATOR:　　　　FACULTY:

108

PROCEDURAL SPECIFICATIONS
MEASUREMENT OF OXYGEN CONCENTRATION

I. Key Performance Elements

Procedural Element (Step)	Description of Satisfactory Performance
1. Selects and gathers appropriate analyzer, accessories	Chooses analyzer appropriate to task, i.e.: a. Clark or galvanic cell for continuous monitoring b. Paramagnetic or thermal conductivity for "spot" analysis Avoids thermal conductivity analyzers in hazardous atmospheres Selects accessories (in-line adapters, etc.) appropriate to task at hand
5. Checks for proper electrical function of analyzer	Confirms electrical power (battery "check") Ensures meter/display/bulb function
8. Slopes analyzer to 100% O_2 or specific known concentration	Checks response for accuracy Adjusts meter/display to appropriate reading Rechecks response to room air Repeats until response verified Replaces/recharges inoperable or defective components if appropriate response not obtained

II. Setting

The student is expected to demonstrate proficiency in the measurement of oxygen concentrations in the following settings: (check those that apply)

☐ Laboratory   ☐ Other (specify)

☐ Clinic

_____

_____

III. Conditions

The student is expected to demonstrate proficiency in the measurement of oxygen concentrations under the following conditions: (check those that apply)

Atmosphere Variables   **Monitoring Variables**

☐ Dry   ☐ Spot checking

☐ Humidified   ☐ Intermittent analysis

☐ Static   ☐ Continuous analysis

☐ Dynamic

Other conditional specifications: _____

_____

_____

IV. Equipment

The student is expected to demonstrate proficiency in the measurement of oxygen concentrations using the following equipment: (check those that apply)

Analyzer Type   **Manufacturer (specify)**

☐ Paramagnetic   _____

☐ Thermal conductivity   _____

☐ Electrochemical (Clark)   _____

☐ Electrochemical (Galvanic   _____
    cell)
☐ Other   _____

V. Outcome Criteria

The oxygen concentration measured and recorded by the student should correspond to that concurrently determined by the evaluator (degree of accuracy ± 2%).

VI. Oral Review Questions

1. Differentiate between the principle of operation, functional characteristics, advantages, disadvantages, and limitations of the following types of oxygen analyzers:
   a. paramagnetic
   b. thermal conductivity
   c. electrochemical (Clark electrode)
   d. electrochemical (Galvanic cell)

2. Of the above categories of analyzers,
   a. which actually measure the partial pressure of oxygen?
   b. which consume oxygen during analysis?
   c. which generate their own current without a power source?
   d. which should not be utilized in a hazardous atmosphere?

3. Describe the anode/cathode reaction typical of a Clark electrode.

4. What other methods are available for the measurement of oxygen concentrations (partial pressure)? What are their advantages/disadvantages?

AEROSOL THERAPY

STUDENT:	DATE:				

PROCEDURE (TASK): AEROSOL/HUMIDITY THERAPY					

SETTING: ☐ LABORATORY ☐ OTHER: (SPECIFY) ☐ CLINIC	SATISFACTORY	UNSATISFACTORY	NOT OBSERVED	NOT APPLICABLE
CONDITIONS (DESCRIBE)				
EQUIPMENT UTILIZED:				

STEPS IN PROCEDURE OR TASK:	SATISFACTORY	UNSATISFACTORY	NOT OBSERVED	NOT APPLICABLE
EQUIPMENT AND PATIENT PREPARATION				
1. Washes hands				
2. Selects, gathers, and assembles appropriate equipment				
3. Verifies, interprets, and evaluates physician's order				
4. Identifies patient, self, and department				
5. Explains procedure and confirms patient understanding				
IMPLEMENTATION AND ASSESSMENT				
6. Adds appropriate solution aseptically and in correct amount				
7. Connects humidifier/aerosol generator to appropriate gas source				
8. Initiates gas flow/aerosol generation				
9. Tests equipment for proper function				
10. Applies modality to patient, ensuring maximum comfort/safety				
11. Ensures gas flow and oxygen concentration appropriate to order/ objectives				
12. Adjusts humidity (aerosol output), temperature appropriate to order/ objectives				
13. Gives additional instructions, where necessary, to maximize therapeutic benefit				
14. Assesses patient response (subjective/objective)				
15. Modifies technique to deal with adverse response				
FOLLOW-UP				
16. Maintains proper equipment function				
17. Records pertinent data in chart and department records				
18. Notifies appropriate personnel				

STUDENT'S COMPREHENSION OF PROCEDURE (SELECT ONE ONLY)

The student demonstrates comprehensive knowledge of basic and advanced concepts beyond requirements of procedure	
The student demonstrates above average understanding of basic concepts applicable to the skill demonstrated	
The student demonstrates adequate knowledge of the essential elements of the task performed	
The student shows limited understanding of essential concepts related to the procedure	
The student has inadequate knowledge of even the basic concepts related to the task at hand	

OUTCOME CRITERIA (WHERE APPLICABLE)

☐ MET	SPECIFY CRITERIA NOT MET AND/OR PERTINENT CONSTRAINTS
☐ NOT MET	
☐ NOT APPL.	

ADDITIONAL COMMENTS

Include errors of omission or commission; if clinical therapeutic procedure emphasize communicative skills (verbal and non-verbal) and effectiveness of patient interaction:

SUMMARY PERFORMANCE EVALUATION AND RECOMMENDATIONS

SETTING	SATISFACTORY	UNSATISFACTORY	SPECIFY DEFICIENCIES
LABORATORY	☐ Can now perform skill under direct clinical supervision	☐ Requires additional laboratory practice	
CLINIC	☐ Ready for minimally supervised application and refinement	☐ Requires additional supervised clinical practice ☐ Complete re-evaluation required ☐ Re-evaluation·minor deficiencies only	

STUDENT: EVALUATOR: FACULTY:

PROCEDURAL SPECIFICATIONS
AEROSOL/HUMIDITY THERAPY

I. Key Performance Elements

Procedural Element (Step)	Description of Satisfactory Performance
6. Adds appropriate solution aseptically and in correct amount	Selects sterile distilled water unless otherwise specified Prevents contamination of internal humidifier/nebulizer components Fills reservoir to specified level
7. Connects humidifier/aerosol generator to appropriate gas source	Selects gas source appropriate for F_1O_2 desired or ordered Selects gas source with appropriate flow/pressure for patient application
9. Test equipment for proper function	Confirms electrical operation, if applicable Confirms operation of relief valves, venturi systems, reservoirs, breathing valves Verifies adequacy of flow Observes, verifies adequacy of bubbling or aerosol production Confirms operation of heating elements Checks patency, operation of continuous feed systems, where applicable Replaces defective or inoperable equipment/components
10. Applies modality to patient, ensuring maximum comfort, safety	Attaches airway apparatus to patient Stabilizes airway apparatus Observes aerosol flow or valve/reservoir action Reassures patient

11. Ensures gas flow and oxygen concentration appropriate to order/objectives

Confirms flow sufficient to (where appropriate):
   a. minimize dead space
   b. prevent reservoir depletion during inspiration
   c. Meet inspiratory flow demands of patient
Confirms gas source/mixing ratios
Measures F_IO_2 where feasible

12. Adjusts humidity (aerosol output), temperature appropriate to order/objectives

Increases/decreases flow or aerosol output to achieve desired humidification or water deposition
Adjusts temperature, where applicable, appropriate to humidification needs

13. Gives additional instructions, where necessary, to maximize therapeutic benefit

Instructs patient in proper breathing pattern
Coaches/reinforces patient cooperation
Ensures proper clearance of secretions

14. Assesses patient response (subjective/objective)

Observes patient for overt changes in breathing pattern
Questions patient regarding comfort
Auscultates thorax (high density aerosol therapy) for indicators of bronchospasm

15. Modifies technique to deal with adverse response

Decreases aerosol density if persistent cough, discomfort
Adjusts temperature if discomfort evident
Discontinues therapy if overt bronchospastic reaction to aerosol develops

II. Setting

The student is expected to demonstrate proficiency in the application of aerosol/humidity therapy in the following settings: (check those that apply)

☐ Laboratory

☐ Clinic

☐ Other (specify)

_____

_____

III. Conditions

The student is expected to demonstrate proficiency in the application of aerosol/humidity therapy under the following conditions: (check those that apply)

Patient Variables

☐ Simulated (peer)

☐ Infant

☐ Adult

☐ Child

Procedure Variables

☐ Intermittent therapy

☐ Continuous therapy

☐ Sputum induction

Other conditional specifications: _____

_____

_____

IV. Equipment

The student is expected to demonstrate proficiency in the application of aerosol/humidity therapy using the following equipment: (check those that apply)

Humidity/Aerosol Generators

☐ Bubble humidifier

☐ Grid humidifier

☐ Wick-type humidifier

☐ Jet nebulizer

☐ Hydronamics nebulizer

☐ Ultrasonic nebulizer

Airway Modality

☐ Simple oxygen modalities

☐ Aerosol mask

☐ T-tube (Brigg's adapter)

☐ Fact tent

☐ Other (specify)

_____

_____

V. Outcome Criteria

Where applicable, the objective(s) of applying humidified gas or aerosol to the airway should be achieved without untoward or adverse patient response.

VI. Oral Review Questions

1. What are the clinical indications for humidity therapy? for aerosol therapy?

2. What potentially beneficial and detrimental physiological effects can result from the application of humidity or aerosol to the airway?

3. What are the common contraindications for aerosol therapy?

4. What objective and subjective means can be used to assess achievement of the desired therapeutic outcomes of aerosol therapy? (Relate patient pathophysiology to intended goals.)

5. What possible alternatives are there to the therapy instituted? What are their advantages/disadvantages?

STUDENT:	DATE:

PROCEDURE (TASK): AEROSOL ENCLOSURES

	SATISFACTORY	UNSATISFACTORY	NOT OBSERVED	NOT APPLICABLE
SETTING: ☐ LABORATORY ☐ OTHER: (SPECIFY) ☐ CLINIC				
CONDITIONS (DESCRIBE)				
EQUIPMENT UTILIZED:				

STEPS IN PROCEDURE OR TASK:

EQUIPMENT AND PATIENT PREPARATION				
1. Washes hands				
2. Selects, gathers, and assembles appropriate equipment				
3. Verifies, interprets, and evaluates physician's order				
4. Identifies patient, self, and department				
5. Explains procedure and confirms patient (family) understanding				
IMPLEMENTATION AND ASSESSMENT				
6. Attaches canopy to frame and secures to bed (crib)				
7. Connects aerosol generator to appropriate gas source				
8. Adds appropriate solution aseptically in correct amount				
9. Tests equipment for proper function				
10. Initiates gas flow and fills enclosure with aerosol				
11. Introduces patient into enclosure				
12. Adjusts gas flow, aerosol output and temperature appropriate to objectives				
13. Ensures patient comfort, canopy fit				
14. Measures F_IO_2, adjusts to prescribed level				
15. Assesses patient response (objective and subjective)				
16. Modifies technique to accommodate response				
17. Follows oxygen safety precautions				
FOLLOW-UP				
18. Maintains proper equipment function				
19. Records pertinent data in chart and department records				
20. Notifies appropriate personnel				

STUDENT'S COMPREHENSION OF PROCEDURE (SELECT ONE ONLY)

The student demonstrates comprehensive knowledge of basic and advanced concepts beyond requirements of procedure	
The student demonstrates above average understanding of basic concepts applicable to the skill demonstrated	
The student demonstrates adequate knowledge of the essential elements of the task performed	
The student shows limited understanding of essential concepts related to the procedure	
The student has inadequate knowledge of even the basic concepts related to the task at hand	

OUTCOME CRITERIA (WHERE APPLICABLE)

☐ MET	SPECIFY CRITERIA NOT MET AND/OR PERTINENT CONSTRAINTS
☐ NOT MET	
☐ NOT APPL.	

ADDITIONAL COMMENTS

Include errors of omission or commission; if clinical therapeutic procedure emphasize communicative skills (verbal and non-verbal) and effectiveness of patient interaction:

SUMMARY PERFORMANCE EVALUATION AND RECOMMENDATIONS

SETTING	SATISFACTORY	UNSATISFACTORY	SPECIFY DEFICIENCIES
LABORATORY	☐ Can now perform skill under direct clinical supervision	☐ Requires additional laboratory practice	
CLINIC	☐ Ready for minimally supervised application and refinement	☐ Requires additional supervised clinical practice ☐ Complete re-evaluation required ☐ Re-evaluation·minor deficiencies only	

STUDENT:　　　　　EVALUATOR:　　　　　FACULTY:

PROCEDURAL SPECIFICATIONS
AEROSOL ENCLOSURES

I. Key Performance Elements

Procedural Element (Step)	Description of Satisfactory Performance
7. Connects aerosol generator to appropriate gas source	Selects gas source corresponding to F_IO_2 ordered
8. Adds appropriate solution aseptically in correct amount	Utilizes sterile distilled water unless otherwise specified Fills reservoir to specified level Ensures function of feed system (where utilized)
9. Tests equipment for proper function	Initiates gas flow Checks for adequate aerosol production Ensures proper gas circulation Checks function of refrigeration/cooling system Rechecks feed system (if utilized) Replaces defective or inoperable equipment/components
10. Initiates gas flow and fills enclosure with aerosol	Sets metering device (if used) at flush Adjusts baffles/dampers if applicable Checks enclosure for appropriate aerosol density
12. Adjusts gas flow, aerosol output, and temperature appropriate to objectives	Sets gas flow sufficient to prevent CO_2 build up (≥ 10 LPM) Adjusts venturi/mixing systems for proper density/flow Measures internal temperature Ensures temperature range within normal (68–74° F)

13. Ensures patient comfort, canopy fit

Maintains patient position away from direct gas flow

Provides reassurance to patient

Folds canopy edge under bedding

Allows for gas evacuation where appropriate (high flow systems)

14. Measures F_IO_2, adjusts to prescribed level

Refer to proficiency evaluation: MEASUREMENT OF OXYGEN CONCENTRATIONS

Adjusts venturi/mixing system to stabilize F_IO_2 at prescribed level

Adds supplement oxygen if necessary

15. Assesses patient response (objective/subjective)

Observes patient for alleviation of symptoms, confirms comfort, allays anxiety

Ensures appropriate monitoring, to include: body weight (for fluid gain); arterial blood gases if oxygen administration

17. Follows oxygen safety precautions

Posts "oxygen-in-use" signs

Removes ignition sources from room

Informs patient (family) and staff of oxygen precautions

18. Maintains proper equipment function

Provides continuous monitoring of F_IO_2 and temperature or

Rechecks F_IO_2, temperature every two hours

Rechecks/replenishes reservoir

Rechecks/readjusts flow/aerosol output

II. Setting

The student is expected to demonstrate proficiency in the application of aerosol enclosures in the following settings: (check those that apply)

☐ Laboratory   ☐ Other

☐ Clinic

_____

_____

III. Conditions

The student is expected to demonstrate proficiency in the application of aerosol enclosures under the following conditions: (check those that apply)

Patient Variables

☐ Simulated (peer/manikin)

☐ Infant

☐ Child

Procedure Variables

☐ Humidity/aerosol only

☐ In combination with oxygen

Other conditional specifications: _____

_____

_____

IV. Equipment

The student is expected to demonstrate proficiency in the application of aerosol enclosures with the following equipment: (check those that apply)

Aerosol Generator

☐ Simple jet nebulizer

☐ High output jet nebulizer

☐ Hydronamics nebulizer

☐ Ultrasonic nebulizer

Cooling System(s)

☐ Ice

☐ Convection cooling

☐ Refrigeration

Reservoir Systems

☐ Large volume reservoir

☐ Float/air lock feed system

☐ Ambient pressure feed system

V. Outcome Criteria

The specified or desired oxygen concentration, temperature, and aerosol density, should be achieved without untoward or adverse patient response.

VI. Oral Review Questions

1. What are the indications and contraindications for high density aerosol therapy?

2. What are the advantages, disadvantages, and limitations of aerosol enclosure therapy as compared to other techniques of aerosol administration?

3. Relate the physical concepts of heat gain/loss to the problems and methods of temperature control within patient enclosures.

4. For the specific apparatus utilized, describe its functional characteristics and principles of operation.

STUDENT:	DATE:				

PROCEDURE (TASK): AEROSOL DRUG ADMINISTRATION

	SATISFACTORY	UNSATISFACTORY	NOT OBSERVED	NOT APPLICABLE
SETTING: ☐ LABORATORY ☐ OTHER: (SPECIFY) ☐ CLINIC				
CONDITIONS (DESCRIBE)				
EQUIPMENT UTILIZED:				

STEPS IN PROCEDURE OR TASK:

	SATISFACTORY	UNSATISFACTORY	NOT OBSERVED	NOT APPLICABLE
EQUIPMENT AND PATIENT PREPARATION				
1. Washes hands				
2. Selects, gathers, and assembles appropriate equipment				
3. Verifies, interprets, and evaluates physician's order				
4. Identifies patient, self, and department				
5. Explains procedure and confirms patient understanding				
IMPLEMENTATION AND ASSESSMENT				
6. Pre-assesses patient (objective and subjective) to establish baseline values				
7. Connects aerosol generator to appropriate gas source				
8. Determines and measures proper dosage of drug/diluent				
9. Adds prescribed drug/diluent to nebulizer chamber				
10. Initiates gas flow				
11. Test equipment for proper function				
12. Properly positions patient				
13. Applies modality to patient, ensuring maximum comfort/safety				
14. Encourages and ensures proper breathing pattern				
15. Adjust gas flow/aerosol output to maximize therapeutic benefit				
16. Checks patient's vital signs, observes response				
17. Modifies technique to deal with adverse patient response				
18. Terminates therapy when complete dosage administered				
19. Encourages patient cough, collects, examines sputum				
20. Conducts post-assessment (objective and subjective), compares to initial measures				
FOLLOW-UP				
21. Maintains/processes equipment				
22. Records pertinent data in chart and department records				
23. Notifies appropriate personnel				

STUDENT'S COMPREHENSION OF PROCEDURE (SELECT ONE ONLY)

The student demonstrates comprehensive knowledge of basic and advanced concepts beyond requirements of procedure	
The student demonstrates above average understanding of basic concepts applicable to the skill demonstrated	
The student demonstrates adequate knowledge of the essential elements of the task performed	
The student shows limited understanding of essential concepts related to the procedure	
The student has inadequate knowledge of even the basic concepts related to the task at hand	

OUTCOME CRITERIA (WHERE APPLICABLE)

☐ MET	SPECIFY CRITERIA NOT MET AND/OR PERTINENT CONSTRAINTS
☐ NOT MET	
☐ NOT APPL.	

ADDITIONAL COMMENTS

Include errors of omission or commission; if clinical therapeutic procedure emphasize communicative skills (verbal and non-verbal) and effectiveness of patient interaction:

SUMMARY PERFORMANCE EVALUATION AND RECOMMENDATIONS

SETTING	SATISFACTORY	UNSATISFACTORY	SPECIFY DEFICIENCIES
LABORATORY	☐ Can now perform skill under direct clinical supervision	☐ Requires additional laboratory practice	
CLINIC	☐ Ready for minimally supervised application and refinement	☐ Requires additional supervised clinical practice ☐ Complete re-evaluation required ☐ Re-evaluation·minor deficiencies only	

STUDENT: EVALUATOR: FACULTY:

PROCEDURAL SPECIFICATIONS
AEROSOL DRUG ADMINISTRATION

I. Key Performance Elements

Procedural Element (Step)	Description of Satisfactory Performance
6. Pre-assesses patient (objective and subjective) to establish baseline values	Refer to proficiency evaluation: PHYSICAL ASSESSMENT, to include: a. assesses vital signs b. auscultates patient's thorax c. measures expiratory flow parameters
7. Connects aerosol generator to appropriate gas source	Selects/ensures F_IO_2 equivalent to that being received
8. Determines and measures proper dosage of drug/ diluent	Checks drug label/concentration Measures drug volume/weight as ordered by physician (utilizes standard order if not specified) Rechecks drug label/concentration Measures diluent volume
11. Tests equipment for proper function	Checks for leaks/obstruction Ensures gas flow (pressure) sufficient to power nebulizer/carry medication Checks for sufficient aerosol output Checks for proper operations of valves, safety systems Replaces inoperative/defective equipment
12. Properly positions patient	Places patient in (semi) Fowler's position Modifies position where necessary

13. Applies modality to patient, ensuring maximum comfort, safety

Attaches mask (airway connector) to patient
Provides for proper fit
Observes aerosol motion
Confirms patient comfort

14. Encourages and ensures proper breathing pattern

Encourages slow, deep inspiration through mouth with breath hold
Modifies instructions if necessary
Reinforces proper pattern throughout treatment

15. Adjusts gas flow/aerosol output to maximize therapeutic benefit

Observes aerosol inhalations/motion
Increases/decreases flow to ensure delivery throughout inspiration
Adjusts aerosol density to accommodate patient's response

16. Checks patient's vital signs, observes response

Refer to proficiency evaluations: VITAL SIGNS, BLOOD PRESSURE
Observes patient for untoward responses

17. Modifies technique to deal with adverse patient response

Decreases aerosol density if severe cough or increase in wheeze, bronchospasm develop
Discontinues therapy if dyspnea, tachycardia, or hypertension develop
Notifies appropriate personnel of untoward patient responses

19. Encourages patient cough, collects, examines sputum

Coaches patient to achieve appropriate cough without deleterious effects:
   a. provides incisional support (post op patients
   b. ensures deep inspiration
   c. solicits maximum effort
   d. repeats/modifies as necessary using adjuncts/techniques appropriate to patient
Refer to proficiency evaluation: COUGHING

20. Conducts postassessment (objective and subjective), compares to initial measures

Measures/ensures stability of vital signs
Measures expiratory flow parameters
Calculates/notes changes in measured pulmonary function
Assures patient comfort

II. Setting

The student is expected to demonstrate proficiency in the administration of drugs by aerosol in the following settings: (check those that apply)

☐ Laboratory

☐ Other (specify)

☐ Clinic

_____

_____

III. Conditions

The student is expected to demonstrate proficiency in the administration of drugs by aerosol under the following conditions: (check those that apply)

Patient Variables

☐ Simulated (peer)

☐ Child

☐ Adult

Procedure Variables

☐ Spontaneous breathing

☐ In conjunction with IPPB

Other conditional specifications: _____

_____

_____

IV. Equipment/Pharmacological Agents

The student is expected to demonstrate proficiency in the administration of drugs by aerosol using the following equipment and pharmacological agents: (check those that apply)

Aerosol Generators

☐ Metered cartridge

☐ Bulb powered nebulizer

☐ Compressed gas powered nebulizer

Airway Modality

☐ Mouthpiece

☐ Mask

☐ Other (specify)

_____

_____

Drug Category

☐ Bronchodilators

☐ Mucolytics

☐ Antibiotics

☐ Other (specify)

Required Agents (specify)

_____

_____

_____

_____

_____

_____

_____

_____

V. Outcome Criteria

The specified or desired effect of the pharmacological agent administered should be achieved without untoward or adverse patient response.

VI. Oral Review Questions

1. What are the advantages, disadvantages, and limitations of drug administration by aerosol as compared to other routes?

2. For the pharmacological agent administered:
   a. what is its normal dosage (weight/volume)?
   b. what is its action?
   c. what are its side effects/hazards?
   d. what contraindications apply to its usage?
   e. how can its desired action be assessed?

HYPERINFLATION THERAPY

STUDENT:	DATE:				

PROCEDURE (TASK): INCENTIVE SPIROMETRY					

SETTING: ☐ LABORATORY ☐ OTHER: (SPECIFY) ☐ CLINIC	SATISFACTORY	UNSATISFACTORY	NOT OBSERVED	NOT APPLICABLE
CONDITIONS (DESCRIBE)				
EQUIPMENT UTILIZED:				

STEPS IN PROCEDURE OR TASK:				
EQUIPMENT AND PATIENT PREPARATION				
1. Washes hands				
2. Selects, gathers, and assembles appropriate equipment				
3. Verifies, interprets, and evaluates physician's order				
4. Identifies patient, self, and department				
5. Explains procedure and confirms patient understanding				
IMPLEMENTATION AND ASSESSMENT				
6. Tests equipment for proper function				
7. Positions patient (and spirometer) properly				
8. Determines patient's inspiratory capacity				
9. Sets appropriate initial goal				
10. Institutes therapy, encourages patient's maximum effort				
11. Observes and evaluates patient response				
12. Readjusts goal appropriate to patient response				
13. Terminates therapy when goal/repetitions achieved				
FOLLOW-UP				
14. Provides instructions to patient on independent use of device				
15. Records pertinent data (progress) in chart and department records				
16. Maintains/processes equipment				
17. Notifies appropriate personnel				

STUDENT'S COMPREHENSION OF PROCEDURE (SELECT ONE ONLY)

The student demonstrates comprehensive knowledge of basic and advanced concepts beyond requirements of procedure	
The student demonstrates above average understanding of basic concepts applicable to the skill demonstrated	
The student demonstrates adequate knowledge of the essential elements of the task performed	
The student shows limited understanding of essential concepts related to the procedure	
The student has inadequate knowledge of even the basic concepts related to the task at hand	

OUTCOME CRITERIA (WHERE APPLICABLE)

☐ MET	SPECIFY CRITERIA NOT MET AND/OR PERTINENT CONSTRAINTS
☐ NOT MET	
☐ NOT APPL.	

ADDITIONAL COMMENTS

Include errors of omission or commission; if clinical therapeutic procedure emphasize communicative skills (verbal and non-verbal) and effectiveness of patient interaction:

SUMMARY PERFORMANCE EVALUATION AND RECOMMENDATIONS

SETTING	SATISFACTORY	UNSATISFACTORY	SPECIFY DEFICIENCIES
LABORATORY	☐ Can now perform skill under direct clinical super-vision	☐ Requires additional laboratory practice	
CLINIC	☐ Ready for min-imally supervised application and refinement	☐ Requires additional supervised clinical practice ☐ Complete re-evaluation required ☐ Re-evaluation·minor deficiencies only	

STUDENT: EVALUATOR: FACULTY:

PROCEDURAL SPECIFICATIONS
INCENTIVE SPIROMETRY

I. Key Performance Elements

Procedural Element (Step)	Description of Satisfactory Performance
6. Tests equipment for proper function	Ensures electrical operation, where applicable Checks function of floats, pistons, or transducer systems for response Replaces defective or inoperable equipment/components
7. Positions patient (and spirometer) properly	Places patient in semi-Fowler's position Assures patient comfort Places and stabilizes metering device in position to assure response (upright)
8. Determines patient's inspiratory capacity	Coaches/instructs patient in performance of inspiratory capacity maneuver Performs trial maneuvers Notes/calculates best performance
9. Sets appropriate initial goal	Sets volume (time/flow) at or near level previously measured
10. Institutes therapy, encourages patient's maximum effort	Identifies set goal and desired repetitions for patient Verbally coaches patient to achieve goal/repetitions/holding time Reinforces achievement of set goals
12. Readjusts goal appropriate to patient response	Increases/decreases goals according to patient achievement and assessment of effort/strength

13. Provides instructions to patient on independent use of device

Explains importance of procedure
Reconfirms patient understanding of technique
Demonstrates documentation system (if applicable)
Sets independent schedule

II. Setting

The student is expected to demonstrate proficiency in the application of incentive spirometry in the following settings: (check those that apply)

☐ Laboratory

☐ Other

☐ Clinic

_____

_____

III. Conditions

The student is expected to demonstrate proficiency in the application of incentive spirometry under the following conditions: (check those that apply)

Patient Variables	Procedure Variables
☐ Simulated (peer)	☐ Continuing supervision
☐ Child	☐ Instruction, independent use with follow-up
☐ Adult	

Other conditional specifications: _____

_____

_____

IV. Equipment

The student is expected to demonstrate proficiency in the application of incentive spirometry using the following equipment: (check those that apply)

Spirometer Type	Manufacturer (specify)
☐ Volumetric, manual	_____
	_____
☐ Volumetric, electronic	_____
	_____
☐ Flow dependent	_____
	_____

V. Outcome Criteria

The goal(s) set and repetitions achieved should be consistent with capabilities of the patient and increase incrementally over the duration of therapy until adequate function is restored and confirmed.

VI. Oral Review Questions

1. What are the clinical indications for incentive spirometry?

2. What potentially beneficial and detrimental physiological effects can result from the application of incentive spirometry?

3. What are the common contraindications for incentive spirometry?

4. What objective and subjective means can be used to assess achievement of the desired therapeutic outcomes of incentive spirometry? (Relate patient pathophysiology to intended goals.)

5. What possible alternatives are there to incentive spirometry? What are their advantages/disadvantages?

STUDENT:		DATE:

PROCEDURE (TASK): INTERMITTENT POSITIVE PRESSURE BREATHING

SETTING: ☐ LABORATORY ☐ OTHER: (SPECIFY) ☐ CLINIC	SATISFACTORY	UNSATISFACTORY	NOT OBSERVED	NOT APPLICABLE
CONDITIONS (DESCRIBE)				
EQUIPMENT UTILIZED:				

STEPS IN PROCEDURE OR TASK:				
EQUIPMENT AND PATIENT PREPARATION	▓	▓	▓	▓
1. Washes hands				
2. Selects, gathers, and assembles appropriate equipment				
3. Verifies, interprets, and evaluates physician's order				
4. Identifies patient, self, and department				
5. Explains procedure and confirms patient understanding				
IMPLEMENTATION AND ASSESSMENT	▓	▓	▓	▓
6. Connects breathing circuit to ventilator				
7. Provides power (pneumatic/electrical) to ventilator				
8. Measures proper dosage of drug/diluent, adds to nebulizer				
9. Cycles ventilator, tests for proper function				
10. Sets initial ventilator values appropriate for patient				
11. Properly positions patient				
12. Pre-assesses patient (objective and subjective)				
13. Applies breathing circuit to patient's airway, initiates therapy				
14. Instructs patient, adjusts ventilator to maintain appropriate parameters				
15. Observes patient response				
16. Modifies technique to accommodate patient's response				
17. Reassesses patient's vital signs, ventilatory parameters				
18. Terminates procedure after appropriate interval				
19. Encourages patient cough, collects, examines sputum				
20. Conducts post-assessment (objective and subjective)				
FOLLOW-UP	▓	▓	▓	▓
21. Maintains/processes equipment				
22. Records pertinent data in chart and department records				
23. Notifies appropriate personnel				

STUDENT'S COMPREHENSION OF PROCEDURE (SELECT ONE ONLY)

The student demonstrates comprehensive knowledge of basic and advanced concepts beyond requirements of procedure	
The student demonstrates above average understanding of basic concepts applicable to the skill demonstrated	
The student demonstrates adequate knowledge of the essential elements of the task performed	
The student shows limited understanding of essential concepts related to the procedure	
The student has inadequate knowledge of even the basic concepts related to the task at hand	

OUTCOME CRITERIA (WHERE APPLICABLE)

☐ MET	SPECIFY CRITERIA NOT MET AND/OR PERTINENT CONSTRAINTS
☐ NOT MET	
☐ NOT APPL.	

ADDITIONAL COMMENTS

Include errors of omission or commission; if clinical therapeutic procedure emphasize communicative skills (verbal and non-verbal) and effectiveness of patient interaction:

SUMMARY PERFORMANCE EVALUATION AND RECOMMENDATIONS

SETTING	SATISFACTORY	UNSATISFACTORY	SPECIFY DEFICIENCIES
LABORATORY	☐ Can now perform skill under direct clinical supervision	☐ Requires additional laboratory practice	
CLINIC	☐ Ready for minimally supervised application and refinement	☐ Requires additional supervised clinical practice ☐ Complete re-evaluation required ☐ Re-evaluation·minor deficiencies only	

STUDENT: EVALUATOR: FACULTY:

PROCEDURAL SPECIFICATIONS
INTERMITTENT POSITIVE PRESSURE BREATHING

I. Key Performance Elements

Procedural Element (Step)	Description of Satisfactory Performance
7. Provides power (pneumatic/ electrical) to ventilator	Selects power source compatible with desired F_IO_2 Ensures unrestricted flow at 50 psi (for pneumatically powered devices)
8. Measures proper dosage of drug/diluent, adds to nebulizer	Determines dosage Confirms drug label/concentration Obtains appropriate volume of drug/diluent aseptically Rechecks drug label/concentration Adds drug/diluent to nebulizer chamber without contamination
9. Cycles ventilator, tests for proper function	Confirms valve action (sensitivity, response) Ensures proper nebulization function Confirms end-inspiratory cycling with test lung or obstruction Replaces defective, inoperative equipment/components
10. Sets initial ventilator values appropriate for patient	Sets initial starting points (for adults) in the following ranges: a. sensitivity of -1 to -2 cm H_2O b. pressure of 12–15 cm H_2O c. flowrate of 30–50 LPM or equivalent

11. Properly positions patient

Places patient (where feasible) in sitting or semi-Fowler's position

12. Pre-assesses patient (objective and subjective)

Measures patient's spontaneous tidal volume, rate, minute ventilation, and inspiratory capacity

Measures patient's expiratory flow parameters (drug-administration)

Measures patient's pulse and blood pressure

Auscultates lung fields

Refer to proficiency evaluations: BEDSIDE VENTILATORY ASSESSMENT, BLOOD PRESSURE, PATIENT ASSESSMENT

13. Applies breathing circuit to patient's airway, initiates therapy

Select appropriate airway attachment

Demonstrate use of airway attachment, explains importance of good seal

Attaches device during patient-expiration

14. Instructs patient, adjusts ventilator to maintain appropriate parameters

Observes for leaks/cycling problems

Obviates or adjusts for leaks/cycling problems

Coaches patient to obtained desired values:
   a. frequency of 10–20 per minute
   b. tidal volume of 7–10 ml/kilogram
   c. inspiratory capacity equal to or exceeding spontaneous inspiratory capacity

15. Observes patient response

Rechecks patient's vital signs

Monitors ventilatory parameters

Reassures patient

16. Modifies technique to accommodate patient's response

Readjusts sensitivity, pressure, flow control to obtain desired values

Discontinues therapy if:
   a. spontaneous IC exceed mechanically augmented IC (for hyperinflation)
   b. frequency or tidal cannot be adjusted to desired range
   c. patient exhibits overt discomfort/signs of hyperventilation

19. Encourages patient cough, collects, examines sputum

Refer to proficiency evaluation: COUGHING

II. Setting

The student will demonstrate proficiency in the application of intermittent positive pressure breathing (IPPB) in the following settings: (check those that apply)

☐ Laboratory

☐ Clinic

☐ Other (specify)

_____

_____

III. Conditions

The student will demonstrate proficiency in the application of IPPB under the following conditions: (check those that apply)

Patient Variables

☐ Simulated (peer)

☐ Child

☐ Adult

Procedure Variables

☐ Hyperinflation only

☐ In combination with drug administration

Other conditional specifications: _____

_____

_____

IV. Equipment

The student will demonstrate proficiency in the application of IPPB using the following equipment: (check those that apply)

Ventilator Type   Manufacturer (specify)

☐ Electrically powered
   (compressor) units   _____

                                         _____

☐ Pneumatically powered,
   sliding alignment valve   _____
   units
                                         _____

☐ Pneumatically powered,   _____
   rotary valve units
                                         _____

☐ Pneumatically powered,   _____
   fluidic units
                                         _____

☐ Other types (specify)   _____

_____   _____

V. Outcome Criteria

When applied to augment lung inflation, the following parameters should be achieved:

Parameter   Desired Value

frequency   10–20/minute (adult)
tidal volume   7–10 ml/kg
inspiratory capacity   equal to or exceeding
                              spontaneous value

When applied to facilitate administration of a pharmacological agent, the desired effect of the drug should be achieved without untoward or adverse patient response.

VI. Oral Review Questions

1. What are the clinical indications for IPPB?

2. What potentially beneficial and detrimental physiological effects can result from performance of IPPB?

3. What are the common contraindications for IPPB?

4. What objective and subjective means can be used to assess achievement of the desired therapeutic outcomes of IPPB? (Relate patient pathophysiology to intended goals.)

5. What possible alternatives are there to IPPB?   What are their advantages/disadvantages?

6. What is the principle of operation and functional characteristics of the equipment utilized for this procedure?

PULMONARY PHYSICAL THERAPY

STUDENT:	DATE:				

PROCEDURE (TASK): BREATHING EXERCISES					

SETTING: ☐ LABORATORY ☐ OTHER: (SPECIFY) ☐ CLINIC	SATISFACTORY	UNSATISFACTORY	NOT OBSERVED	NOT APPLICABLE
CONDITIONS (DESCRIBE)				
EQUIPMENT UTILIZED:				

STEPS IN PROCEDURE OR TASK:				
EQUIPMENT AND PATIENT PREPARATION				
1. Washes hands				
2. Selects, gathers, and assembles appropriate equipment				
3. Verifies, interprets, and evaluates physician's order				
4. Identifies patient, self, and department				
5. Explains procedure and confirms patient understanding				
IMPLEMENTATION AND ASSESSMENT				
6. Positions patient				
7. Demonstrates procedure on self				
8. Observes/palpates applicable muscle activity				
9. Instructs patient to coordinate applicable muscle activity				
10. Applies inspiratory resistance to applicable muscle group				
11. Encourages slow, forceful inspiration, passive exhalation				
12. Observes and corrects common errors				
13. Repeats procedure as indicated/tolerated				
FOLLOW-UP				
14. Demonstrates methods of self-application				
15. Provides reinforcement for conformance				
16. Returns patient to comfortable position				
17. Records pertinent data in chart and departmental records				
18. Maintains/processes equipment				
19. Notifies appropriate personnel				

STUDENT'S COMPREHENSION OF PROCEDURE (SELECT ONE ONLY)

The student demonstrates comprehensive knowledge of basic and advanced concepts beyond requirements of procedure	
The student demonstrates above average understanding of basic concepts applicable to the skill demonstrated	
The student demonstrates adequate knowledge of the essential elements of the task performed	
The student shows limited understanding of essential concepts related to the procedure	
The student has inadequate knowledge of even the basic concepts related to the task at hand	

OUTCOME CRITERIA (WHERE APPLICABLE)

☐ MET	SPECIFY CRITERIA NOT MET AND/OR PERTINENT CONSTRAINTS
☐ NOT MET	
☐ NOT APPL.	

ADDITIONAL COMMENTS

Include errors of omission or commission; if clinical therapeutic procedure emphasize communicative skills (verbal and non-verbal) and effectiveness of patient interaction:

SUMMARY PERFORMANCE EVALUATION AND RECOMMENDATIONS

SETTING	SATISFACTORY	UNSATISFACTORY	SPECIFY DEFICIENCIES
LABORATORY	☐ Can now perform skill under direct clinical supervision	☐ Requires additional laboratory practice	

CLINIC	☐ Ready for minimally supervised application and refinement	☐ Requires additional supervised clinical practice
		  ☐ Complete re-evaluation required
		  ☐ Re-evaluation·minor deficiencies only	

STUDENT: EVALUATOR: FACULTY:

PROCEDURAL SPECIFICATIONS
BREATHING EXERCISES

I. Key Performance Elements

Procedural Element (Step)	Description of Satisfactory Performance
6. Positions patient	Places patient (where possible) in semi-Fowler's position Provides back and head support Ensure flexion/support of knees, relaxation of abdominal muscles Refer to proficiency evaluation: PATIENT POSITIONING
7. Demonstrates procedure on self	Provides example of coordinated breathing cycle Demonstrate applicable muscle activity by hand placement
8. Observes/palpates applicable muscle activity	Places hands over applicable muscle group Notes nature and magnitude of existing motion
9. Instructs patient to coordinate applicable muscle activity	Encourages slow inspiration Focuses patient attention on applicable muscle group Encourages coordinated muscle use (inspiration)
10. Applies inspiratory resistance to applicable muscle group	Applies incremental pressure during inspiration Encourages patient to "push out" against resistance Repeats/modifies instructions as necessary
12. Observes and corrects common errors	Prevents forceful exhalation Encourages slow and even respiratory pattern Minimizes use of accessory muscles

14. Demonstrates methods of self-application

Positions patient's hands over applicable muscle group

Applies incremental pressure over patient's hands during inspiration

Coaches patient to do the same

Confirms patient's conformance

II. Setting

The student is expected to demonstrate proficiency in the application of breathing exercises in the following settings: (check those that apply)

☐ Laboratory

☐ Clinic

☐ Other (specify)

_____

_____

III. Conditions

The student is expected to demonstrate proficiency in the application of breathing exercises under the following conditions: (check those that apply)

Patient Variables

☐ Simulated (peer)

☐ Child

☐ Adult

Procedure Variables

☐ Diaphragmatic breathing

☐ Segmental breathing

Other conditional specifications: _____

_____

_____

IV. Equipment

Applicable equipment includes that pertaining to the proficiency evaluation PATIENT POSITIONING.

V. Outcome Criteria

After initial instruction and reinforcement, the patient should be able to demonstrate appropriate use of the applicable muscle group and properly coordinate the inspiratory and expiratory phases of breathing, to the satisfaction of the evaluator.

VI. Oral Review Questions

1. Differentiate between the goals/purposes of breathing exercises for the following patient groups:
   a. postoperative chest or abdominal surgery
   b. chronic obstructive pulmonary disease

2. What potentially detrimental physiological effects can result from the following common patient errors in breathing
   a. forceful exhalation?
   b. rapid breathing?
   c. overuse of accessory muscles?

3. What objective and subjective means can be used to assess achievement of the desired therapeutic outcomes of breathing exercises? (Relate patient pathophysiology to intended goals.)

4. What possible alternatives are there to the application of breathing exercises? What are their advantages and disadvantages?

STUDENT:		DATE:			

PROCEDURE (TASK): COUGHING					

SETTING: ☐ LABORATORY ☐ OTHER: (SPECIFY) ☐ CLINIC	SATISFACTORY	UNSATISFACTORY	NOT OBSERVED	NOT APPLICABLE
CONDITIONS (DESCRIBE)				
EQUIPMENT UTILIZED:				

STEPS IN PROCEDURE OR TASK:				
EQUIPMENT AND PATIENT PREPARATION				
1. Washes hands				
2. Selects, gathers, and assembles appropriate equipment				
3. Verifies, interprets, and evaluates physician's order				
4. Identifies patient, self, and department				
5. Explains procedure and confirms patient understanding				
IMPLEMENTATION AND ASSESSMENT				
6. Positions patient				
7. Pre-assesses patient				
8. Instructs patient in effective use of diaphragm				
9. Demonstrates cough phases on self				
10. Provides incisional support (postoperative)				
11. Encourages deep inspiration, inspiratory hold				
12. Assures forceful contraction of abdominal muscles				
13. Observes and corrects common errors				
14. Modifies technique as appropriate to patient				
15. Reassesses patient				
16. Repeats procedure as indicated/tolerated				
17. Examines (collects) sputum				
FOLLOW-UP				
18. Provides reinforcement for conformance				
19. Returns patient to comfortable position				
20. Records pertinent data in chart and department records				
21. Maintains/processes equipment				
22. Notifies appropriate personnel				

STUDENT'S COMPREHENSION OF PROCEDURE (SELECT ONE ONLY)

The student demonstrates comprehensive knowledge of basic and advanced concepts beyond requirements of procedure	
The student demonstrates above average understanding of basic concepts applicable to the skill demonstrated	
The student demonstrates adequate knowledge of the essential elements of the task performed	
The student shows limited understanding of essential concepts related to the procedure	
The student has inadequate knowledge of even the basic concepts related to the task at hand	

OUTCOME CRITERIA (WHERE APPLICABLE)

☐ MET	SPECIFY CRITERIA NOT MET AND/OR PERTINENT CONSTRAINTS
☐ NOT MET	
☐ NOT APPL.	

ADDITIONAL COMMENTS

Include errors of omission or commission; if clinical therapeutic procedure emphasize communicative skills (verbal and non-verbal) and effectiveness of patient interaction:

SUMMARY PERFORMANCE EVALUATION AND RECOMMENDATIONS

SETTING	SATISFACTORY	UNSATISFACTORY	SPECIFY DEFICIENCIES
LABORATORY	☐ Can now perform skill under direct clinical super- vision	☐ Requires additional laboratory practice	
CLINIC	☐ Ready for min- imally supervised application and refinement	☐ Requires additional supervised clinical practice ☐ Complete re- evaluation required ☐ Re-evaluation·minor deficiencies only	

STUDENT: EVALUATOR: FACULTY:

PROCEDURAL SPECIFICATIONS
COUGHING

I. Key Performance Elements

Procedural Element (Step)	Description of Satisfactory Performance
3. Verifies, interprets, and evaluates physician's order	Identifies any hazards/ contraindications to the procedure Ascertains need for modifications in technique
6. Positions patient	Places patient (where possible) in semi-Fowler's position Assures forward flexion of trunk Modifies position according to need/tolerance
7. Pre-assesses patient	Auscultates thorax for manifestations of excessive secretions, airway obstruction Refer to proficiency evaluation: PATIENT ASSESSMENT
8. Instructs patient in effective use of diaphragm	Refer to proficiency evaluation: BREATHING EXERCISES
9. Demonstrates cough phases on self	Provides example of coordinated cough cycle, to include: a. deep inspiration b. inspiratory hold c. forceful expulsion Repeats demonstration as necessary
10. Provides incisional support (postoperative)	Uses pillow or flat of hands over incisional site Demonstrates application of self-splinting technique

12. Assures forceful contraction of abdominal muscles

Places hands over abdomen
Applies pressure during expiration
Encourages forceful contraction

13. Observes and corrects common errors

Ensures deep inspiration
Discourages "hacking," throat clearance
Confirms glottic closure
Encourages forceful expulsion

14. Modifies technique as appropriate to patient

Uses "huff" technique where indicated
Modifies force of expulsion where danger of airway closure
Enhances productivity by aerosol administration
Stimulates cough reflex by tracheal pressure or suction catheter

15. Reassesses patient

Auscultates thorax for manifestations of excessive secretions, airway obstruction
Notes changes from initial assessment

17. Examines (collects) sputum

Isolates sputum in appropriate container
Notes color, consistency, and amount of secretions

II. Setting

The student is expected to demonstrate proficiency in the application of coughing methods in the following settings: (check those that apply)

☐ Laboratory

☐ Other (specify)

☐ Clinic

_____

_____

III. Conditions

The student is expected to demonstrate proficiency in the application of coughing methods under the following conditions: (check those that apply)

Patient Variables	Procedure Variables

☐ Simulated (peer)   ☐ Sputum collection

☐ Postoperative patient   ☐ Tracheobronchial aspiration

☐ COPD patient   ☐ In conjunction with aerosol

Other conditional specifications: _____

_____

_____

IV. Equipment

Applicable equipment includes that pertaining to the proficiency evaluations PATIENT POSITIONING, PATIENT ASSESSMENT, BREATHING EXERCISES, AEROSOL THERAPY, and TRACHEO-BRONCHIAL ASPIRATION.

V. Outcome Criteria

Where manifestations of excessive secretions and/or airway obstruction are noted on pre-assessment of the patient, post-assessment should reveal tangible improvement. Moreover, after initial instruction and reinforcement, the (alert) patient should be able to demonstrate an effective cough cycle, to the satisfaction of the evaluator.

VI. Oral Review Questions

1. For each of the three major phases of a voluntary cough cycle, specify the conditions which could compromise a patient's ability to generate an effective cough.

2. What are the contraindications for the voluntary production of a forceful expulsive cough?

3. What objective and subjective means can be used to assess achievement of the desired therapeutic outcomes of cough? (Relate patient pathophysiology to intended goals.)

4. What alternative methods of airway clearance are available for:
   a. unconscious or obtunded patients?
   b. patients with an artificial airway?
   c. refractory airway obstruction?

STUDENT:	DATE:

PROCEDURE (TASK): POSTURAL DRAINAGE AND PERCUSSION

	SATISFACTORY	UNSATISFACTORY	NOT OBSERVED	NOT APPLICABLE
SETTING: ☐ LABORATORY ☐ OTHER: (SPECIFY) ☐ CLINIC				
CONDITIONS (DESCRIBE)				
EQUIPMENT UTILIZED:				

STEPS IN PROCEDURE OR TASK:	SATISFACTORY	UNSATISFACTORY	NOT OBSERVED	NOT APPLICABLE
EQUIPMENT AND PATIENT PREPARATION	▒	▒	▒	▒
1. Washes hands				
2. Selects, gathers, and assembles appropriate equipment				
3. Verifies, interprets, and evaluates physician's order				
4. Identifies patient, self, and department				
5. Explains procedure and confirms patient understanding				
IMPLEMENTATION AND ASSESSMENT	▒	▒	▒	▒
6. Pre-assesses patient				
7. Instructs (demonstrates) patient in diaphragmatic breathing, segmental expansion and coughing				
8. Positions patient for segmental/lobar drainage				
9. Assesses patient response/tolerance				
10. Modifies position to accommodate patient's response				
11. Encourages maintenance of proper breathing pattern				
12. Performs percussion over properly identified area				
13. Perform vibration over correct area during expiration				
14. Encourages and assists patient with cough/expectoration				
15. Examines (collects) sputum				
16. Maintains position for appropriate time interval				
17. Repositions patient and repeats procedure as indicated/tolerated				
18. Returns patient to comfortable position				
19. Reassesses patient				
FOLLOW-UP	▒	▒	▒	▒
20. Provides reinforcement for conformance				
21. Records pertinent data in chart and department records				
22. Maintains/processes equipment				
23. Notifies appropriate personnel				

STUDENT'S COMPREHENSION OF PROCEDURE (SELECT ONE ONLY)

The student demonstrates comprehensive knowledge of basic and advanced concepts beyond requirements of procedure	
The student demonstrates above average understanding of basic concepts applicable to the skill demonstrated	
The student demonstrates adequate knowledge of the essential elements of the task performed	
The student shows limited understanding of essential concepts related to the procedure	
The student has inadequate knowledge of even the basic concepts related to the task at hand	

OUTCOME CRITERIA (WHERE APPLICABLE)

☐ MET	SPECIFY CRITERIA NOT MET AND/OR PERTINENT CONSTRAINTS
☐ NOT MET	
☐ NOT APPL.	

ADDITIONAL COMMENTS

Include errors of omission or commission; if clinical therapeutic procedure emphasize communicative skills (verbal and non-verbal) and effectiveness of patient interaction:

SUMMARY PERFORMANCE EVALUATION AND RECOMMENDATIONS

SETTING	SATISFACTORY	UNSATISFACTORY	SPECIFY DEFICIENCIES
LABORATORY	☐ Can now perform skill under direct clinical supervision	☐ Requires additional laboratory practice	
CLINIC	☐ Ready for minimally supervised application and refinement	☐ Requires additional supervised clinical practice ☐ Complete re-evaluation required ☐ Re-evaluation·minor deficiencies only	

STUDENT: EVALUATOR: FACULTY:

PROCEDURAL SPECIFICATIONS
POSTURAL DRAINAGE AND PERCUSSION

I. Key Performance Elements

Procedural Element (Step)	Description of Satisfactory Performance
3. Verifies, interprets, and evaluates physician's order	Refer to proficiency evaluation: MEDICAL RECORDS Utilizes history, physical, radiology report to localize lesion Identifies any hazards/contraindications to technique utilized
6. Pre-assesses patient	Refer to proficiency evaluations: VITAL SIGNS, BLOOD PRESSURE, PATIENT ASSESSMENT
7. Instructs (demonstrates) patient in diaphragmatic breathing, segmental expansion, and coughing	Refer to proficiency evaluations: BREATHING EXERCISES, COUGHING
8. Positions patient for segmental/lobar drainage	Selects position appropriate to lesion location Refer to proficiency evaluation: PATIENT POSITIONING
9. Assesses patient response/tolerance	Questions patient as to comfort Observes patient for untoward responses Refer to proficiency evaluations: VITAL SIGNS, BLOOD PRESSURE

10. Modifies position to accommodate patient's response

Elevates/repositions patient if complaint of pain, dyspnea, dizziness, or changes in vital signs occur

Discontinues therapy if intolerable pain, severe dyspnea, or unstable vital signs develop

11. Encourages maintenance of proper breathing pattern

Coaches patient to breath slowly, deeply

Ensures proper I/E ratio

12. Performs percussion over properly identified area

Identifies boundaries, defines area margins for percussion

Strikes chest wall for appropriate time interval with cupped hands with good rate/rhythm and over defined boundaries

Assures patient comfort

13. Performs vibrations over correct area during expiration

Identifies boundaries, defines area margins for vibration

Places flat of hand over area to be vibrated

Coaches patient to exhale

Tenses arm muscles, applies vibratory motion

14. Encourages and assists pa- with cough/expectoration

Refer to proficiency evaluation: COUGHING

15. Examines (collects) sputum

Aspirates secretions (if necessary)

Isolates sputum in appropriate container

Notes color, consistency, and amount of secretions

19. Reassesses patient

Refer to proficiency evaluations: VITAL SIGNS, PATIENT ASSESSMENT

Confirms stability of vital signs

II. Setting

The student is expected to demonstrate proficiency in the application of postural drainage and percussion in the following settings: (check those that apply)

□ Laboratory   □ Other (specify)

□ Clinic

_____

_____

III. Conditions

The student is expected to demonstrate proficiency in the application of postural drainage and percussion under the following conditions: (check those that apply)

Patient Variables	Procedure Variables
□ Simulated (peer)	□ Conscious, cooperative patient
□ Infant	□ Obtunded patient
□ Child	□ Patient receiving ventilatory support
□ Adult	

Other conditional specifications: _____

_____

_____

IV. Equipment

Applicable equipment includes that pertaining to the proficiency evaluations PATIENT POSITIONING, PATIENT ASSESSMENT, BREATHING EXERCISES, TRACHEOBRONCHIAL ASPIRATION, and COUGHING.

In addition, the student is expected to demonstrate proficiency in the application of percussion and vibration techniques using the following equipment:

□ Electronically powered vibrator/percussor

□ Gas powered vibrator/percussor

V. Outcome Criteria

Where manifestations of excessive secretions and/or airway obstruction are noted on pre-assessment of the patient, postassessment should reveal tangible improvement.

VI. Oral Review Questions

1. What are the clinical indications for postural drainage and percussion?

2. What potentially beneficial and detrimental physiological effects can result from performance of postural drainage and percussion?

3. What are the common contraindications for postural drainage and percussion?

4. What objective and subjective means can be used to assess achievement of the desired therapeutic outcomes of postural drainage and percussion? (Relate patient pathophysiology to intended goals.)

5. What possible alternatives are there to postural drainage and percussion? What are their advantages/disadvantages?

EMERGENCY PROCEDURES

STUDENT:	DATE:

PROCEDURE (TASK): CARDIOPULMONARY RESUSCITATION (ADULT)

SETTING: ☐ LABORATORY ☐ OTHER: (SPECIFY) ☐ CLINIC	SATISFACTORY	UNSATISFACTORY	NOT OBSERVED	NOT APPLICABLE
CONDITIONS (DESCRIBE)				
EQUIPMENT UTILIZED:				
STEPS IN PROCEDURE OR TASK:				
ASSESSMENT				
1. Establishes unresponsiveness				
2. Summons help				
3. Opens airway/establishes breathlessness				
4. Identifies arrhythmia (if monitored)				
IMPLEMENTATION (BASIC LIFE SUPPORT)				
5. Administers four quick breaths				
6. Clears airway (obstruction)				
7. Establishes pulselessness				
8. Initiates chest compressions/maintains ventilation				
9. Checks for return of pulse and spontaneous breathing				
10. Maintains effective ventilation/compression ratio				
IMPLEMENTATION (ADVANCED LIFE SUPPORT)				
11. Selects, inserts and secures airway adjunct				
12. Selects and applies manual ventilator (oxygenates)				
13. Checks for return of pulse and spontaneous breathing				
14. Aspirates airway				
15. Continues support as indicated				
FOLLOW-UP				
16. Provides post-resuscitative support/care				
17. Maintains/processes equipment				
18. Records pertinent data in chart and departmental records				

STUDENT'S COMPREHENSION OF PROCEDURE (SELECT ONE ONLY)

The student demonstrates comprehensive knowledge of basic and advanced concepts beyond requirements of procedure	
The student demonstrates above average understanding of basic concepts applicable to the skill demonstrated	
The student demonstrates adequate knowledge of the essential elements of the task performed	
The student shows limited understanding of essential concepts related to the procedure	
The student has inadequate knowledge of even the basic concepts related to the task at hand	

OUTCOME CRITERIA (WHERE APPLICABLE)

☐ MET	SPECIFY CRITERIA NOT MET AND/OR PERTINENT CONSTRAINTS
☐ NOT MET	
☐ NOT APPL.	

ADDITIONAL COMMENTS

Include errors of omission or commission; if clinical therapeutic procedure emphasize communicative skills (verbal and non-verbal) and effectiveness of patient interaction:

SUMMARY PERFORMANCE EVALUATION AND RECOMMENDATIONS

SETTING	SATISFACTORY	UNSATISFACTORY	SPECIFY DEFICIENCIES
LABORATORY	☐ Can now perform skill under direct clinical supervision	☐ Requires additional laboratory practice	

CLINIC	☐ Ready for minimally supervised application and refinement	☐ Requires additional supervised clinical practice
		    ☐ Complete re-evaluation required
		    ☐ Re-evaluation·minor deficiencies only	

STUDENT: EVALUATOR: FACULTY:

172

PROCEDURAL SPECIFICATIONS
CARDIOPULMONARY RESUSCITATION (ADULT)

I. Key Performance Elements

Procedural Element (Step)	Description of Satisfactory Performance

1. Establishes unresponsiveness	Shakes patient's shoulder
	Shouts "Are You OK?"
	Proceeds if no response
	   (Elapsed time of 4 to 10
	   seconds)

3. Opens airway/establishes breathlessness	Hyperextends patient's neck
	Thrusts chin/jaw forward
	Tilts ear over patient's
	   airway, listens for
	   breath sounds
	Observes chest for excursions
	   (Elapsed time of 7 to 15
	   seconds)

4. Identifies arrhythmia (if monitored)	Differentiates between arti-
	   facts and true arrhythmias
	Distinguishes between minor
	   and lethal arrhythmias
	   (Elapsed time of 7 to 15
	   seconds)

5. Administers four quick breaths	Fills own lungs
	Ensures adequate seal
	Maintains airway position
	Inflates patient's lungs with
	   four repetitive expirations
	Observes chest excursions
	   (Elapsed time of 10 to 20
	   seconds)

6. Clears airway (obstruction)	Repositions airway
	Reattempts ventilation
	If unsuccessful, provides four
	   back blows
	If unsuccessful, provides four
	   abdominal or chest thrusts
	If unsuccessful, uses finger
	   sweep to check for foreign
	   bodies
	Reattempts ventilation
	Repeats sequence until suc-
	   cessful (Elapsed time 33
	   to 52 seconds)

7. Establishes pulselessness

Slides fingers to side of larynx
Palpates carotid pulse
Proceeds if no discernible pulse (Elapsed time, without airway obstruction, of 15 to 30 seconds)

8. Initiates chest compressions/ maintains ventilation

Positions self to side of patient's thorax
Checks sternal landmarks
Places heel of hand over lower third of sternum
Keeps arms straight and elbows locked
Exerts firm, heavy downward force on chest, depressing sternum $1\frac{1}{2}$ to 2 inches
Utilizes slight compression pause
Releases pressure
Repeats at rate of 60 per minute
Ventilates at appropriate intervals:
   a. 2 breaths/15 compressions if alone
   b. 1 breath/15 compressions with assistance
Maintains 60 compressions/ 10 ventilations per minute (Elapsed time, without airway obstruction, of 69 to 96 seconds)

9. Checks for return of pulse and spontaneous breathing

Palpates carotid pulse
Checks pupil dilation/ reactivity
Observes for spontaneous chest excursions
Observes for spontaneous motion
Proceeds if no indication of response

11. Selects, inserts, and secures airway adjunct	Chooses airway of proper size Positions patient Inserts airway Confirms airway patency Secures airway Refer to proficiency evaluation: EMERGENCY ENDOTRACHEAL INTUBATION
12. Selects and applies manual ventilator (oxygenates)	Connects ventilator to 100% oxygen source, approximately metered Confirms ventilator function Connects ventilator to airway Checks for leaks/obstructions Maintains airway position (mask) Confirms adequate ventilation
14. Aspirates airway	Refer to proficiency evaluation: TRACHEOBRONCHIAL ASPIRATION

II. Setting

The student is expected to demonstrate proficiency in cardio-pulmonary resuscitation of the adult in the following settings: (check those apply)

☐ Laboratory   ☐ Other (specify)

☐ Clinic

_____

_____

III. Conditions

The student is expected to demonstrate proficiency in the cardiopulmonary resuscitation of the adult under the following conditions: (check those that apply)

Patient Variables	Procedure Variables
☐ Simulated (recording manikin)	☐ Unobstructed airway
☐ Adult, unmonitored	☐ Obstructed airway
☐ Adult, monitored	☐ Artificial airway in place

Other conditional specifications: _____

_____

_____

IV. Equipment

The student is expected to demonstrate proficiency in the cardiopulmonary resuscitation of the adult using the following equipment: (check those that apply)

Airway Adjuncts	Manual Ventilators
☐ Oropharyngeal airways	☐ Self-inflating bag/valve system (specify)
☐ Nasopharyngeal airways	
☐ Assorted masks	_____
☐ Orotracheal tubes	☐ Gas powered resuscitator (specify)
☐ Nasotracheal tubes	_____
☐ Esophageal obturator	☐ Anesthesia bag/valve system

Other equipment specifications: _____

_____

_____

V. Outcome Criteria

Simulated performance of adult basic life support on an approved recording manikin must correspond to the most recent standards established by the American Heart Association.

VI. Oral Review Questions

1. Under what specific circumstances must the standard procedure for establishing an airway be altered? How is it altered?

2. What special considerations in the performance of cardiopulmonary resuscitation on an adult apply in the following situations:
   a. water submersion (drowning)?
   b. accident cases?
   c. electrical shock?

3. What are the major hazards of cardiopulmonary resuscitation? What are the major pitfalls to successful resuscitation?

4. For each of the following categories of drugs used during Advanced Cardiac Life Support (ACLS), (1) cite a representative pharmacological agent, (2) describe its indication(s), action, and side effects/hazards, and (3) identify its recommended dosage/infusion rate for adults in cardiopulmonary arrest:
   a. anti-arrhythmatic agents
   b. cardiotonic/vasoactive agents
   c. blood/fluid buffers
   d. diuretic agents

5. Describe the postresuscitative special care management considerations applicable to the following organ systems:
   a. respiratory system
   b. cardiovascular system
   c. renal system
   d. central nervous system
   e. gastrointestinal system

6. Describe the principle of operation and functional characteristics of the manual ventilator(s) used to provide advanced life support.

STUDENT:	DATE:

PROCEDURE (TASK):CARDIOPULMONARY RESUSCITATION (Infant/Child)

SETTING: ☐ LABORATORY ☐ OTHER: (SPECIFY) ☐ CLINIC	SATISFACTORY	UNSATISFACTORY	NOT OBSERVED	NOT APPLICABLE
CONDITIONS (DESCRIBE)				
EQUIPMENT UTILIZED:				

STEPS IN PROCEDURE OR TASK:				
ASSESSMENT				
1. Establishes unresponsiveness				
2. Summons help				
3. Opens airway/establishes breathlessness				
4. Identifies arrhythmia (if monitored)				
IMPLEMENTATION (BASIC LIFE SUPPORT)				
5. Administers four quick breaths				
6. Clears airway (obstruction)				
7. Establishes pulselessness				
8. Initiates chest compressions/maintains ventilation				
9. Checks for return of pulse and spontaneous breathing				
10. Maintains effective ventilation/compression ratio				
IMPLEMENTATION (ADVANCED LIFE SUPPORT)				
11. Selects, inserts, and secures airway adjunct				
12. Selects and applies manual ventilator (oxygenates)				
13. Checks for return of pulse and spontaneous breathing				
14. Aspirates airway				
15. Continues support as indicated				
FOLLOW-UP				
16. Provides post-resuscitative support/care				
17. Maintains/processes equipment				
18. Records pertinent data in chart and departmental records				

STUDENT'S COMPREHENSION OF PROCEDURE (SELECT ONE ONLY)

The student demonstrates comprehensive knowledge of basic and advanced concepts beyond requirements of procedure	
The student demonstrates above average understanding of basic concepts applicable to the skill demonstrated	
The student demonstrates adequate knowledge of the essential elements of the task performed	
The student shows limited understanding of essential concepts related to the procedure	
The student has inadequate knowledge of even the basic concepts related to the task at hand	

OUTCOME CRITERIA (WHERE APPLICABLE)

☐ MET	SPECIFY CRITERIA NOT MET AND/OR PERTINENT CONSTRAINTS
☐ NOT MET	
☐ NOT APPL.	

ADDITIONAL COMMENTS

Include errors of omission or commission; if clinical therapeutic procedure emphasize communicative skills (verbal and non-verbal) and effectiveness of patient interaction:

SUMMARY PERFORMANCE EVALUATION AND RECOMMENDATIONS

SETTING	SATISFACTORY	UNSATISFACTORY	SPECIFY DEFICIENCIES
LABORATORY	☐ Can now perform skill under direct clinical supervision	☐ Requires additional laboratory practice	
CLINIC	☐ Ready for minimally supervised application and refinement	☐ Requires additional supervised clinical practice ☐ Complete re-evaluation required ☐ Re-evaluation·minor deficiencies only	

STUDENT:　　　　　EVALUATOR:　　　　　FACULTY:

PROCEDURAL SPECIFICATIONS
CARDIOPULMONARY RESUSCITATION (INFANT/CHILD)

I. Key Performance Elements

Procedural Element (Step)	Description of Satisfactory Performance
1. Establishes unresponsiveness	Shakes patient's shoulder Proceeds if no response (Elapsed time of 3 to 5 seconds)
3. Opens airway/establishes breathlessness	Tilts patient's head/neck Thrusts chin/jaw forward Avoids soft tissue compression under jaw Tilts ear over patient's airway, listens for breath sounds Observes chest for excursions (Elapsed time of 6 to 10 seconds)
4. Identifies arrhythmia (if monitored)	Differentiates between artifacts and true arrhythmias Distinguishes between minor and lethal arrhythmias (Elapsed time of 6 to 10 seconds)
5. Administers four quick breaths	Fills own lungs Ensures adequate seal (mouth/nose for infant) Maintains airway position Inflates patient's lungs with four repetitive expirations sufficient to make chest rise Observes chest excursions (Elapsed time of 9 to 15 seconds)

6. Clears airway (obstruction)

Repositions airway
Reattempts ventilation
Differentiates between in-
     fectious and foreign body
     causes of obstruction
If foreign body likely,
     provides four back blows
If unsuccessful, provides
     four chest thrusts
If unsuccessful, opens mouth,
     thrusts jaw forward,
     displaces tongue,
     visualizes airway
Removes visible foreign body
     with finger
Reattempts ventilation
Repeats sequence until
     successful (Elapsed time
     of 30 to 47 seconds)

7. Establishes pulselessness

Palpates brachial pulse
Proceeds if no discernible
     pulse (Elapsed time,
     without airway obstruction,
     of 14 to 25 seconds)

8. Initiates chest compressions/
   maintains ventilations

Positions self to side of
     patient's thorax
Checks sternal landmarks
Places three fingers (heel
     of hand) over middle of
     sternum
Keeps arms straight and
     elbows locked
Exerts firm, downward force
     on chest, depressing
     sternum $\frac{1}{2}$ to 1 inch
     (infant), 1 to 1$\frac{1}{2}$ inch
     (child)
Utilizes slight compression
     pause
Releases pressure
Repeats at rate of 100 per
     minute (infant), 80 per
     minute (child)
Ventilates at appropriate
     intervals:
     a. 1 breath every 3
        seconds (infant)
     b. 1 breath every 4
        seconds (child)

	Maintains compression to respiration ratio of 5:1 (Elapsed time, without airway obstruction, of 44 to 55 seconds)
9. Checks for return of pulse and spontaneous breathing	Palpates brachial pulse Checks pupil dilation/ reactivity Observes for spontaneous chest excursions Observes for spontaneous motion Proceeds if no indication of response
11. Selects, inserts, and secures airway adjunct	Chooses airway of proper size Positions patient Inserts airway Confirms airway patency Secures airway Refer to proficiency evaluation: EMERGENCY ENDO-TRACHEAL INTUBATION
12. Selects and applies manual ventilator (oxygenates)	Connects ventilator to 100% oxygen source, appropriately metered Confirms ventilator function Connects ventilator to airway Checks for leaks/obstruction Maintains airway position (mask) Confirms adequate ventilation
14. Aspirates airway	Refer to proficiency evaluation: TRACHEOBRONCHIAL ASPIRATION Monitors heart rate for bradycardia

II. Setting

The student is expected to demonstrate proficiency in cardio-pulmonary resuscitation of the infant/child in the following setting: (check those that apply)

☐ Laboratory

☐ Clinic

☐ Other (specify)

_____

_____

III. Conditions

The student is expected to demonstrate proficiency in the cardiopulmonary resuscitation of the infant/child under the following conditions: (check those that apply)

Patient Variables	Procedure Variables
☐ Simulated (simple manikin)	☐ Unobstructed airway
☐ Simulated (recording manikin)	☐ Obstructed airway
☐ Newborn	☐ Artificial airway in place
☐ Infant	
☐ Child	

Other conditional specifications: _____

_____

_____

IV. Equipment

The student is expected to demonstrate proficiency in the cardiopulmonary resuscitation of the infant/child using the following equipment: (check those that apply)

Airway Adjuncts	Manual Ventilators
☐ Oropharyngeal airways	☐ Self-inflating bag/valve system (specify)
☐ Assorted masks	
☐ Orotracheal tubes	_____
☐ Nasotracheal tubes	☐ Gas powered resuscitator (specify)
	_____
	☐ Anesthesia bag/valve system

Other equipment specifications: _____

_____

_____

V. Outcome Criteria

Simulated performance of basic life support for the infant or child on an approved manikin (simple or recording) must correspond to the most recent standards established by the American Heart Association.

VI. Oral Review Questions

1. Differentiate between the common causes and appropriate management of airway obstruction in the neonate, infant, and child.

2. Specify the recommended sizes for (1) oral airway, (2) endotracheal tube, and (3) suction catheter in the following infants/children:
   a. 1,000 gram or less newborn
   b. 1,250 to 2,500 gram newborn
   c. 3,000 grams or more newborn
   d. 18 month old infant
   e. 5 year old child

3. Differentiate between the resuscitative treatment of the following two categories of neonates:
   a. respirations depressed or absent, heart rate greater than 100 beats per minute
   b. Respirations depressed or absent, heart rate less than 100 beats per minute

STUDENT:		DATE:				

PROCEDURE (TASK): EMERGENCY ENDOTRACHEAL INTUBATION

	SATISFACTORY	UNSATISFACTORY	NOT OBSERVED	NOT APPLICABLE
SETTING: ☐ LABORATORY ☐ OTHER: (SPECIFY) ☐ CLINIC				
CONDITIONS (DESCRIBE)				
EQUIPMENT UTILIZED:				
STEPS IN PROCEDURE OR TASK:				
EQUIPMENT AND PATIENT PREPARATION				
1. Washes hands				
2. Selects, gathers, and assembles appropriate equipment				
3. Explains procedure and confirms patient understanding				
4. Provides for sedation (where necessary)				
IMPLEMENTATION				
5. Positions patient				
6. Clears airway				
7. Anesthetizes airway				
8. Hyperoxygenates patient				
9. Inserts laryngoscope into oropharynx				
10. Exposes, lifts epiglottis and visualizes cords				
11. Inserts endotracheal tube through vocal cords				
12. Inflates tube cuff				
13. Provides ventilation, hyperoxygenation				
14. Auscultates chest for symmetrical ventilation				
FOLLOW-UP				
15. Marks proximal end of tube				
16. Secures and stabilizes tube				
17. Aspirates trachea, bronchi				
18. Provides post-intubation care/support				
19. Provides for follow-up chest radiograph				
20. Maintains/processes equipment				
21. Records pertinent data in chart and departmental records				
22. Notifies appropriate personnel				

STUDENT'S COMPREHENSION OF PROCEDURE (SELECT ONE ONLY)

The student demonstrates comprehensive knowledge of basic and advanced concepts beyond requirements of procedure	
The student demonstrates above average understanding of basic concepts applicable to the skill demonstrated	
The student demonstrates adequate knowledge of the essential elements of the task performed	
The student shows limited understanding of essential concepts related to the procedure	
The student has inadequate knowledge of even the basic concepts related to the task at hand	

OUTCOME CRITERIA (WHERE APPLICABLE)

☐ MET	SPECIFY CRITERIA NOT MET AND/OR PERTINENT CONSTRAINTS
☐ NOT MET	
☐ NOT APPL.	

ADDITIONAL COMMENTS

Include errors of omission or commission; if clinical therapeutic procedure emphasize communicative skills (verbal and non-verbal) and effectiveness of patient interaction:

SUMMARY PERFORMANCE EVALUATION AND RECOMMENDATIONS

SETTING	SATISFACTORY	UNSATISFACTORY	SPECIFY DEFICIENCIES
LABORATORY	☐ Can now perform skill under direct clinical supervision	☐ Requires additional laboratory practice	
CLINIC	☐ Ready for minimally supervised application and refinement	☐ Requires additional supervised clinical practice ☐ Complete re-evaluation required ☐ Re-evaluation•minor deficiencies only	

STUDENT: EVALUATOR: FACULTY:

PROCEDURAL SPECIFICATIONS
EMERGENCY ENDOTRACHEAL INTUBATION

I. Key Performance Elements

Procedural Element (Step)	Description of Satisfactory Performance

2. Selects, gathers, and assembles appropriate equipment	Checks/confirms operation of key equipment, including:
	  a. laryngoscope bulb(s)
	  b. suction source
	  c. oxygen source
	  d. tube cuff(s)
	Selects appropriate size endotracheal tube(s)
	Lubricates endotracheal tube(s)
	Inserts stylet into tube(s)

5. Positions patient	Places patient in supine position Provides shoulder support Flexes head at neck Extends atlanto-occipital joint Moves chin up and back
6. Clears airway	Removes all visible forms of obstruction, including dentures Suctions oropharynx
7. Anesthetizes airway	Pulls tongue forward Sprays topical anesthetic agent over mouth, pharynx, laryngeal inlet
8. Hyperoxygenates patient	Hyperinflates patient's lungs with resuscitation bag and mask Uses 100% oxygen Oxygenates for minimum of one minute

9. Inserts laryngoscope into oropharynx

Holds laryngoscope in left hand
Opens mouth with right hand
Inserts blade tip along right side of tongue
Advances blade to base of tongue, displaces to the left
Avoids striking teeth

10. Exposes, lifts epiglottis and visualizes cords

Moves blade to center of pharynx
Places blade tip in appropriate position:
a. curved blade in vallecula
b. straight blade below base of epiglottis
Displaces epiglottis with lifting motion
Exposes glottis

11. Inserts endotracheal tube through vocal cords

Introduces tube tip into right corner of mouth
Passes tube along axis intersecting with line of laryngoscope blade
Passes tube tip through cords until cuff just disappears from sight

17. Aspirates trachea, bronchi

Refer to proficiency evaluation: TRACHEOBRONCHIAL ASPIRATIONS
Checks aspirated fluids for pH

18. Provides post-intubation care/support

Maintains appropriate cuff volume/pressure
Provides for adequate airway humidification
Provides necessary bronchial hygiene regimen
Provides ventilatory support (where necessary)
Refer to proficiency evaluations: CUFF MANAGEMENT, AEROSOL/ HUMIDITY THERAPY, TRACHEOBRONCHIAL ASPIRATION, VENTILATOR PREPARATION, and APPLICATION

II. Setting

The student is expected to demonstrate proficiency in emergency endotracheal intubation in the following settings: (check those that apply)

☐ Laboratory

☐ Clinic

☐ Other (specify)

_____

_____

III. Conditions

The student is expected to demonstrate proficiency in emergency endotracheal intubation under the following conditions: (check those that apply)

Patient Variables

☐ Simulated (Adult manikin)

☐ Simulated (Infant manikin)

☐ Infant

☐ Child

☐ Adult

Procedure Variables

☐ In combination with cardiopulmonary resuscitation

☐ In preparation for instituting mechanical ventilation

☐ In preparation for operative (general) anesthesia

Method Variables

☐ Orotracheal intubation

☐ Nasotracheal intubation

Other conditional specifications: _____

_____

_____

IV. Equipment

The student is expected to demonstrate proficiency in emergency endotracheal intubation with the following equipment: (check those that apply)

Laryngoscope Blades

☐ Curved (MacIntosh)

☐ Straight (Miller)

Accessories

☐ Magill forceps

☐ Stylet

☐ Pharyngeal suction tip (Yankauer)

Endotracheal Tubes

☐ Adult, high volume, low pressure gas-filled cuffs

☐ Adult, self-inflating foam-filled cuffs

☐ Infant/child, cuffless

☐ Other (specify): _____

_____

Additional equipment (where required) includes that applicable to the proficiency evaluations CARDIOPULMONARY RESUSCITATION, CUFF MANAGEMENT, AEROSOL/HUMIDITY THERAPY, TRACHEOBRONCHIAL ASPIRATION, and VENTILATOR PREPARATION AND APPLICATION

V. Outcome Criteria

After completion of the procedure, the endotracheal tube must be secured and stabilized in the appropriate position as verified by auscultation, chest radiograph, and/or fiberoptic laryngoscopy. All appropriate and necessary post-intubation support must be adequately provided according to need.

VI. Oral Review Questions

1. What equipment should be included in an emergency endotracheal intubation tray or kit?

2. Describe the characteristics of an ideal adult endotracheal tube, as established by the Z-79 Committee for Anesthesia Equipment of the United States Standards Institute.

3. Differentiate between the indications for, advantages of, disadvantages of, limitations of, and procedures for orotracheal and nasotracheal intubation.

4. Identify the common complications (and methods for minimizing their occurrence) of the following stages of intubation management:

    a. during the procedure itself
    b. while the tube is in place
    c. during and after extubation (late complications)

5. What special considerations apply to the intubation of infants and small children?

6. What other ways are available to establish an unobstructed airway during an emergency? What are their advantages, disadvantages, limitations, and hazards?

AIRWAY CARE

STUDENT:	DATE:				

PROCEDURE (TASK): TRACHEOBRONCHIAL ASPIRATION

SETTING: ☐ LABORATORY ☐ OTHER: (SPECIFY) ☐ CLINIC

CONDITIONS (DESCRIBE)

EQUIPMENT UTILIZED:

STEPS IN PROCEDURE OR TASK:	SATISFACTORY	UNSATISFACTORY	NOT OBSERVED	NOT APPLICABLE
EQUIPMENT AND PATIENT PREPARATION				
1. Selects, gathers, and assembles appropriate equipment				
2. Identifies patient, self, and department				
3. Explains procedure and confirms patient understanding				
IMPLEMENTATION AND ASSESSMENT				
4. Assesses patient/patient airway				
5. Hyperoxygenates and hyperinflates patient				
6. Washes hands				
7. Adjusts suction to appropriate level				
8. Positions patient				
9. Dons sterile glove(s)				
10. Pours (sterile) water into (sterile) bowl				
11. Attaches sputum trap to suction source				
12. Attaches catheter to suction source				
13. Reassures patient				
14. Inserts catheter until resistance met				
15. Withdraws catheter 1 to 2 centimeters				
16. Applies intermittent suction, rotates/withdraws catheter				
17. Clears catheter, repeats as necessary				
18. Hyperoxygenates and hyperinflates patient				
19. Reassesses patient/patient airway				
20. Reassures patient				
FOLLOW-UP				
21. Restores patient to prior status				
22. Maintains/processes equipment				
23. Records pertinent data in chart and departmental records				
24. Notifies appropriate personnel				

STUDENT'S COMPREHENSION OF PROCEDURE (SELECT ONE ONLY)

The student demonstrates comprehensive knowledge of basic and advanced concepts beyond requirements of procedure	
The student demonstrates above average understanding of basic concepts applicable to the skill demonstrated	
The student demonstrates adequate knowledge of the essential elements of the task performed	
The student shows limited understanding of essential concepts related to the procedure	
The student has inadequate knowledge of even the basic concepts related to the task at hand	

OUTCOME CRITERIA (WHERE APPLICABLE)

☐ MET	SPECIFY CRITERIA NOT MET AND/OR PERTINENT CONSTRAINTS
☐ NOT MET	
☐ NOT APPL.	

ADDITIONAL COMMENTS

Include errors of omission or commission; if clinical therapeutic procedure emphasize communicative skills (verbal and non-verbal) and effectiveness of patient interaction:

SUMMARY PERFORMANCE EVALUATION AND RECOMMENDATIONS

SETTING	SATISFACTORY	UNSATISFACTORY	SPECIFY DEFICIENCIES
LABORATORY	☐ Can now perform skill under direct clinical supervision	☐ Requires additional laboratory practice	
CLINIC	☐ Ready for minimally supervised application and refinement	☐ Requires additional supervised clinical practice ☐ Complete re-evaluation required ☐ Re-evaluation·minor deficiencies only	

STUDENT: EVALUATOR: FACULTY:

PROCEDURAL SPECIFICATIONS
TRACHEOBRONCHIAL ASPIRATION

I. Key Performance Elements

Procedural Element (Step)	Description of Satisfactory Performance
4. Assesses patient/patient airway	Establishes baseline vital signs Auscultates trachea/bronchi for manifestations of excessive secretions Refer to proficiency evaluations: VITAL SIGNS, PATIENT ASSESSMENT
5. Hyperoxygenates and hyper-inflates patient	Employs manual resuscitator for spontaneous breathing patients Utilizes sigh mode for patient on mechanical ventilator Provides 100% oxygen for minimum of one minute
7. Adjusts suction to appropriate level	Selects appropriate therapeutic range: a. 120–150 mmHg for adults b. 80–120 mmHg for children c. 60–80 mmHg for infants Confirms operation of suction equipment
8. Positions patient	Uses semi-Fowler's position (where possible) Rotates head/neck for selective bronchial insertion
14. Inserts catheter until resistance met	Lubricates catheter (where necessary) Keeps thumbport vent open If oro/nasal route: a. opens mouth/extends tongue b. instructs patient to breathe slowly/deeply

       c. passes catheter through glottis during inspiration

       d. assures tracheal placement

16. Applies intermittent suction, rotates/withdraws catheter

Controls suction with thumb-port vent

Rotates 360° between fingers

Limits application of suction to 10–15 seconds

Discontinues procedure if adverse cardiovascular response observed

22. Maintains/processes equipment

Discards disposable supplies

Removes sputum trap, seals, labels, and forwards

II. Setting

The student is expected to demonstrate proficiency in the application of tracheobronchial aspiration in the following settings: (check those that apply)

☐ Laboratory

☐ Clinic

☐ Other (specify)

_____

_____

III. Conditions

The student is expected to demonstrate proficiency in the application of tracheobronchial aspiration under the following conditions: (check those that apply)

Patient Variables

☐ Simulated (manikin)

☐ Infant

☐ Child

☐ Adult

Procedure Variables

☐ Orotracheal aspiration

☐ Nasotracheal aspiration

☐ Aspiration through an artificial airway

☐ In conjunction with sterile sputum collection

Other conditional specifications: _____

_____

_____

IV. Equipment

The student is expected to demonstrate proficiency in the application of tracheobronchial aspiration with the following equipment: (check those that apply)

Vacuum Source | Catheter Type(s)

☐ Mobile electric suction pump | ☐ Standard straight-tipped, beveled edge
☐ Mobile pneumatic aspirator | ☐ Ring-tipped

☐ Central piped vacuum system | ☐ Angle-tipped (Coudé)

V. Outcome Criteria

Where evidence of excessive secretions is noted on preassessment, tracheobronchial aspiration should result in a tangible improvement in airway status, as confirmed by auscultation. When applied to obtain a sputum sample, the specimen obtained must be of sufficient volume for analysis and maintained in a sterile state.

VI. Oral Review Questions

1. Identify the common complications of tracheobronchial aspiration; for each hazard identified, describe its manifestations and specify a method of minimizing or eliminating its detrimental effect upon the patient.

2. How does one determine the appropriate size catheter to be used with an artificial airway? Why is this relationship important?

3. Describe the design characteristics and rationale for the use of:
    a. ring-tipped catheters
    b. angle-tipped catheters

4. What alternative procedures are available for clearance of inspissated or impacted tracheobronchial secretions? What are their advantages, disadvantages, limitations, and hazards?

STUDENT:		DATE:				

PROCEDURE (TASK): CUFF MANAGEMENT

SETTING: ☐ LABORATORY ☐ OTHER: (SPECIFY) ☐ CLINIC	SATISFACTORY	UNSATISFACTORY	NOT OBSERVED	NOT APPLICABLE
CONDITIONS (DESCRIBE)				
EQUIPMENT UTILIZED:				

STEPS IN PROCEDURE OR TASK:	SATISFACTORY	UNSATISFACTORY	NOT OBSERVED	NOT APPLICABLE
EQUIPMENT AND PATIENT PREPARATION	▒	▒	▒	▒
1. Washes hands				
2. Selects, gathers, and assembles appropriate equipment				
3. Verifies, interprets, and evaluates physician's order				
4. Identifies patient, self, and department				
5. Explains procedure and confirms patient's understanding				
IMPLEMENTATION	▒	▒	▒	▒
6. Aspirates oro/hypopharynx				
7. Deflates cuff				
8. Connects pressure gauge to cuff inflation line				
9. Connects syringe to "Y" fitting				
10. Provides inspiratory positive pressure				
11. Auscultates over cuff site				
12. Inflates cuff to minimal occluding volume				
13. Deflate cuff until minimal leak, observes pressure				
14. Secures cuff inflation inlet (valve)				
15. Reassures patient				
FOLLOW-UP	▒	▒	▒	▒
16. Maintains/processes equipment				
17. Records pertinent data in chart and departmental records				
18. Notifies appropriate personnel				

STUDENT'S COMPREHENSION OF PROCEDURE (SELECT ONE ONLY)

The student demonstrates comprehensive knowledge of basic and advanced concepts beyond requirements of procedure	
The student demonstrates above average understanding of basic concepts applicable to the skill demonstrated	
The student demonstrates adequate knowledge of the essential elements of the task performed	
The student shows limited understanding of essential concepts related to the procedure	
The student has inadequate knowledge of even the basic concepts related to the task at hand	

OUTCOME CRITERIA (WHERE APPLICABLE)

☐ MET	SPECIFY CRITERIA NOT MET AND/OR PERTINENT CONSTRAINTS
☐ NOT MET	
☐ NOT APPL.	

ADDITIONAL COMMENTS

Include errors of omission or commission; if clinical therapeutic procedure emphasize communicative skills (verbal and non-verbal) and effectiveness of patient interaction:

SUMMARY PERFORMANCE EVALUATION AND RECOMMENDATIONS

SETTING	SATISFACTORY	UNSATISFACTORY	SPECIFY DEFICIENCIES
LABORATORY	☐ Can now perform skill under direct clinical super-vision	☐ Requires additional laboratory practice	
CLINIC	☐ Ready for min-imally supervised application and refinement	☐ Requires additional supervised clinical practice ☐ Complete re-evaluation required ☐ Re-evaluation·minor deficiencies only	

STUDENT: EVALUATOR: FACULTY:

PROCEDURAL SPECIFICATIONS
CUFF MANAGEMENT

I. Key Performance Elements

Procedural Element (Step)	Description of Satisfactory Performance
6. Aspirates oro/hypopharynx	Opens mouth/extends patient's tongue Passes catheter into oro/hypopharynx Applies intermittent suction Repeats as necessary Disposes catheter (avoids subsequent use in trachea)
12. Inflates cuff to minimal occluding volume	Slowly injects air into pilot line Simultaneously auscultates over cuff site Confirms absence of inspiratory gas leakage
13. Deflates cuff until minimal leak, observes pressure	Slowly withdraws gas with syringe Simultaneously auscultates over cuff site Stops gas withdrawal when audible leak occurs, at lowest possible pressure (less than 25 mmHg)
17. Records pertinent data in chart and departmental records	Notes cuff pressure and volume required for minimal leak
18. Notifies appropriate personnel	Informs nurse/physician of problems: a. cuff leakage b. incremental increases in volume/pressure

II. Setting

The student is expected to demonstrate proficiency in the application of cuff management procedures in the following settings: (check those that apply)

☐ Laboratory   ☐ Other (specify)

☐ Clinic

_____

_____

III. Conditions

The student is expected to demonstrate proficiency in the application of cuff management procedures under the following conditions: (check those that apply)

Patient Variables   Procedure Variables

☐ Simulated (manikin)   ☐ Cuff used to protect lower
                                     airway only
☐ Child   ☐ Cuff used to provide
                                     positive pressure
☐ Adult   ventilation

Other conditional specifications: _____

_____

_____

IV. Equipment

The student is expected to demonstrate proficiency in the application of cuff management procedures, using the following equipment: (check those that apply)

Manometer Type(s)   Cuff Type(s)

☐ Aneroid   ☐ Gas-filled

☐ Mercurial   ☐ Foam-filled

Additional equipment includes that applicable to the proficiency evaluation TRACHEOBRONCHIAL ASPIRATION.

V. Outcome Criteria

When cuff inflation is used to provide a seal for positive pressure, a minimal occluding volume or minimal leak should be obtained at cuff pressures less than 25 mmHg. Protection of the lower airway from aspiration of oral/gastric secretions should be confirmed by a negative methylene blue test.

VI. Oral Review Questions

1. What is the physiological rationale for low lateral tracheal wall pressures with artificial airway cuffs?

2. Differentiate between the advantages and disadvantages of Minimal Occluding Volume and Minimal Leak Technique as methods of cuff management in patients receiving positive pressure ventilation. What two conditions are desirable goals in adjusting cuff pressure/volume?

3. In order to obtain a minimal leak on a patient receiving positive pressure ventilation, you find (from shift to shift) that it is necessary to incrementally increase cuff pressure and volume. What is the potential cause of this problem? What would you recommend to the physician?

4. A patient receiving mechanical ventilation via a cuffed tracheostomy tube with an inner cannula exhibits a sudden rise in airway pressure. You remove the patient from the ventilator and unsuccessfully try to ventilate her with a manual resuscitator. What steps (in what order) would you follow to deal with this emergency airway obstruction?

STUDENT:		DATE:				

PROCEDURE (TASK): TRACHEOSTOMY CARE

	SATISFACTORY	UNSATISFACTORY	NOT OBSERVED	NOT APPLICABLE
SETTING: ☐ LABORATORY ☐ OTHER: (SPECIFY) ☐ CLINIC				
CONDITIONS (DESCRIBE)				
EQUIPMENT UTILIZED:				

STEPS IN PROCEDURE OR TASK:	SATISFACTORY	UNSATISFACTORY	NOT OBSERVED	NOT APPLICABLE
EQUIPMENT AND PATIENT PREPARATION				
1. Selects, gathers, and assembles appropriate equipment				
2. Verifies, interprets, and evaluates physician's order				
3. Identifies patient, self, and department				
4. Explains procedure and confirms patient understanding				
IMPLEMENTATION AND ASSESSMENT				
5. Positions patient				
6. Washes hands				
7. Dons sterile gloves				
8. Removes ties, stoma dressing				
9. Cleans stoma				
10. Removes inner cannula, cleans/rinses				
11. Replaces inner cannula, stabilizes				
12. Places new sterile dressing around tube				
13. Resecures tube with clean ties				
14. Rechecks tube position/stability				
15. Auscultates chest/cuff site				
16. Reassures patient				
FOLLOW-UP				
17. Restores patient to prior status				
18. Maintains/processes equipment				
19. Records pertinent data in chart and departmental records				
20. Notifies appropriate personnel				

STUDENT'S COMPREHENSION OF PROCEDURE (SELECT ONE ONLY)

The student demonstrates comprehensive knowledge of basic and advanced concepts beyond requirements of procedure	
The student demonstrates above average understanding of basic concepts applicable to the skill demonstrated	
The student demonstrates adequate knowledge of the essential elements of the task performed	
The student shows limited understanding of essential concepts related to the procedure	
The student has inadequate knowledge of even the basic concepts related to the task at hand	

OUTCOME CRITERIA (WHERE APPLICABLE)

☐ MET	SPECIFY CRITERIA NOT MET AND/OR PERTINENT CONSTRAINTS
☐ NOT MET	
☐ NOT APPL.	

ADDITIONAL COMMENTS

Include errors of omission or commission; if clinical therapeutic procedure emphasize communicative skills (verbal and non-verbal) and effectiveness of patient interaction:

SUMMARY PERFORMANCE EVALUATION AND RECOMMENDATIONS

SETTING	SATISFACTORY	UNSATISFACTORY	SPECIFY DEFICIENCIES
LABORATORY	☐ Can now perform skill under direct clinical supervision	☐ Requires additional laboratory practice	
CLINIC	☐ Ready for minimally supervised application and refinement	☐ Requires additional supervised clinical practice ☐ Complete re-evaluation required ☐ Re-evaluation minor deficiencies only	

STUDENT: EVALUATOR: FACULTY:

PROCEDURAL SPECIFICATIONS
TRACHEOSTOMY CARE

I. Key Performance Elements

Procedural Element (Step)	Description of Satisfactory Performance
5. Positions patient	Provides support to patient's shoulders Aligns head, neck, thorax Extends neck to access tracheal stoma
8. Removes ties, stoma dressing	Ensures stability of tube Uses assistance (where necessary)
9. Cleans stoma	Uses hydrogen peroxide or equivalent Cleans stoma gently with sterile swabs Observes stoma site for signs of inflammation, infection, bleeding, or subcutaneous emphysema
10. Removes inner cannula, cleans/rinses	Unlocks cannula, removes Replaces cannula with temporary Scrubs inside of cannula with brush, peroxide Rinses cannula in sterile water
13. Resecures tube with clean ties	Tightens ties sufficiently to prevent tube displacement Uses square knot to secure ties
14. Rechecks tube position/stability	Ensures proper alignment Confirms tracheal placement Confirms stability
15. Auscultates chest/cuff site	Confirms symmetrical ventilation Confirms appropriate cuff inflation Refer to proficiency evaluation: CUFF MANAGEMENT

II. Setting

The student is expected to demonstrate proficiency in tracheostomy care in the following settings: (check those that apply)

☐ Laboratory   ☐ Other (specify)

☐ Clinic

_____

_____

III. Conditions

The student is expected to demonstrate proficiency in tracheostomy care under the following conditions: (check those that apply)

Patient Variables

☐ Simulated (manikin)

☐ Child

☐ Adult

Other conditional specifications: _____

Procedure Variables

☐ Wound/tube care only

☐ Change of tracheostomy tube

_____

_____

IV. Equipment

The student is expected to demonstrate proficiency in tracheostomy care with the following equipment: (check those that apply)

Tube Types

☐ Metal (permanent)

☐ Standard plastic polymer, cuffed

☐ Tracheostomy button

Cannula

☐ Without inner cannula

☐ With inner cannula

☐ Fenestrated cannula

V. Outcome Criteria

After completion of tracheostomy care, the cleaned (replaced) tube should be stable, properly positioned in the stoma/trachea with (where applicable) the cuff properly inflated.

VI. Oral Review Questions

1. Differentiate between the indications for, advantages, disadvantages, limitations, and hazards of tracheostomy versus oro/nasotracheal intubation.

2. For each of the patients below, identify the appropriate size (range) tracheostomy tube (French size and/or external diameter):
   a. six month old infant
   b. four year old child
   c. eight year old child
   d. twelve year old child
   e. female adult, average size
   f. male adult, average size

3. Why is it recommended that tracheostomy tubes not be changed until 2–3 days after establishing the stoma? What methods can be used to facilitate tracheostomy tube replacement? What action should be taken if a tracheostomy tube becomes dislodged and cannot be immediately replaced?

4. Describe the clinical manifestations, potential sequelae, and methods of prevention or rectification of the following common complications of tracheostomy:
   a. cannulation of mainstem bronchus
   b. cuff dislodgement/tube occlusion
   c. misplacement of tube in subcutaneous tissues
   d. occlusion of tube against tracheal wall
   e. ruptured tube cuff
   f. tracheal wall erosion/fistula
   g. tube obstruction with inspissated secretions

STUDENT:		DATE:

PROCEDURE (TASK): ENDOTRACHEAL EXTUBATION

	SATISFACTORY	UNSATISFACTORY	NOT OBSERVED	NOT APPLICABLE
SETTING: ☐ LABORATORY ☐ OTHER: (SPECIFY) ☐ CLINIC				
CONDITIONS (DESCRIBE)				
EQUIPMENT UTILIZED:				

STEPS IN PROCEDURE OR TASK:

EQUIPMENT AND PATIENT PREPARATION				
1. Selects, gathers, and assembles appropriate equipment				
2. Verifies, interprets, and evaluates physician's order				
3. Identifies patient, self, and department				
4. Explains procedure and confirms patient understanding				
IMPLEMENTATION AND ASSESSMENT				
5. Confirms ventilatory status/airway function				
6. Positions patient				
7. Aspirates trachea, oro/hypopharynx				
8. Hyperoxygenates and hyperinflates patient				
9. Unsecures tube				
10. Deflates cuff				
11. Passes suction catheter beyond tube tip				
12. Instructs patient to breath deeply				
13. Remove tube/catheter while applying suction				
14. Encourages patient to cough				
15. Reassures patient				
FOLLOW-UP				
16. Provides appropriate humidification and oxygenation				
17. Monitors and observes patient response				
18. Maintains/processes equipment				
19. Records pertinent data in chart and departmental record				
20. Notifies appropriate personnel				

STUDENT'S COMPREHENSION OF PROCEDURE (SELECT ONE ONLY)

The student demonstrates comprehensive knowledge of basic and advanced concepts beyond requirements of procedure	
The student demonstrates above average understanding of basic concepts applicable to the skill demonstrated	
The student demonstrates adequate knowledge of the essential elements of the task performed	
The student shows limited understanding of essential concepts related to the procedure	
The student has inadequate knowledge of even the basic concepts related to the task at hand	

OUTCOME CRITERIA (WHERE APPLICABLE)

☐ MET	SPECIFY CRITERIA NOT MET AND/OR PERTINENT CONSTRAINTS
☐ NOT MET	
☐ NOT APPL.	

ADDITIONAL COMMENTS

Include errors of omission or commission; if clinical therapeutic procedure emphasize communicative skills (verbal and non-verbal) and effectiveness of patient interaction:

SUMMARY PERFORMANCE EVALUATION AND RECOMMENDATIONS

SETTING	SATISFACTORY	UNSATISFACTORY	SPECIFY DEFICIENCIES
LABORATORY	☐ Can now perform skill under direct clinical supervision	☐ Requires additional laboratory practice	
CLINIC	☐ Ready for minimally supervised application and refinement	☐ Requires additional supervised clinical practice ☐ Complete re-evaluation required ☐ Re-evaluation·minor deficiencies only	

STUDENT: EVALUATOR: FACULTY:

PROCEDURAL SPECIFICATIONS
ENDOTRACHEAL EXTUBATION

I. Key Performance Elements

Procedural Element (Step)	Description of Satisfactory Performance
1. Selects, gathers, and assembles appropriate equipment	Prepares and confirms operation of: a. suction equipment b. aerosol/humidity equipment c. oxygen therapy equipment Ensures availability of intubation/tracheostomy trays
5. Confirms ventilatory status, airway function	Ensures adequacy of forceful expiration Confirms function of upper airway protective reflexes (methylene blue test) Refer to proficiency evaluation: BEDSIDE VENTILATORY ASSESSMENT
6. Positions patient	Uses semi-Fowler's position Aligns head, neck, trachea Provides shoulder support Extends neck
7. Aspirates trachea, oro/hypopharynx	Refer to proficiency evaluation: TRACHEOBRONCHIAL ASPIRATION
13. Removes tube/catheter while applying suction	Waits until peak of inspiration Applies suction to catheter Gently and quickly removes tube
14. Encourages patient to cough	Refer to proficiency evaluation: COUGHING

16. Provides appropriate humidification and oxygenation

Ensures oxygen concentration equal to or exceeding pre-extubation levels
Provides supplementary humidity/aerosol appropriate to needs

17. Monitors and observes patient response

Monitors vital signs
Auscultates thorax for manifestations of excessive secretions
Confirms satisfactory ventilatory parameters
Obtains arterial blood gas
Assesses blood gases
Refer to proficiency evaluations: VITAL SIGNS, PATIENT ASSESSMENT, BEDSIDE VENTILATORY ASSESSMENT, ARTERIAL BLOOD GAS SAMPLING, and ARTERIAL BLOOD GAS ANALYSIS

II. Setting

The student is expected to demonstrate proficiency in endotracheal extubation in the following settings: (check those that apply)

☐ Laboratory

☐ Clinic

☐ Other (specify)

_____

_____

III. Conditions

The student is expected to demonstrate proficiency in endotracheal extubation under the following conditions: (check those that apply)

Patient Variables

☐ Simulated (manikin)

☐ Infant

☐ Child

☐ Adult

Procedure Variables

☐ Orotracheal tube

☐ Nasotracheal tube

☐ Tracheostomy tube

Other conditional specifications: _____

_____

_____

IV. Equipment

The equipment applicable to endotracheal extubation is that utilized for the following proficiency evaluations: BEDSIDE VENTILATORY ASSESSMENT, TRACHEOBRONCHIAL ASPIRATION, AEROSOL/HUMIDITY THERAPY, OXYGEN THERAPY, ARTERIAL BLOOD GAS SAMPLING, and ARTERIAL BLOOD GAS ANALYSIS.

V. Outcome Criteria

After extubation, the patient should be able to maintain, without undo work, adequate ventilation and oxygenation, as determined by the appropriate methods of assessment. Moreover, the patient should demonstrate adequate airway clearance by coughing and be able to swallow fluids without aspiration.

VI. Oral Review Questions

1. What physiological and/or mechanical criteria can be used to assess a patient's readiness for removal of an endotracheal airway? What values of these criteria would favor extubation?

2. Describe the method(s) whereby the efficacy of a patient's upper airway protective reflexes can be assessed.

3. Differentiate among the hazards of extubating a patient with (a) a tracheostomy tube, (b) an orotracheal tube, and (c) a nasotracheal tube.

4. What common complications should one be alert to during the early post-extubation phase of airway management? What are the clinical manifestations of these complications? What response is necessary to alleviate or reverse their effect?

DIAGNOSTIC AND
ASSESSMENT PROCEDURES

STUDENT:		DATE:				

PROCEDURE (TASK): BEDSIDE VENTILATORY ASSESSMENT

	SATISFACTORY	UNSATISFACTORY	NOT OBSERVED	NOT APPLICABLE
SETTING: ☐ LABORATORY ☐ OTHER: (SPECIFY) ☐ CLINIC				
CONDITIONS (DESCRIBE)				
EQUIPMENT UTILIZED:				

STEPS IN PROCEDURE OR TASK:

	SATISFACTORY	UNSATISFACTORY	NOT OBSERVED	NOT APPLICABLE
EQUIPMENT AND PATIENT PREPARATION				
1. Washes hands				
2. Selects, gathers, and assembles appropriate equipment				
3. Verifies, interprets, and evaluates physician's order				
4. Identifies patient, self, and department				
5. Explains procedure and confirms patient understanding				
IMPLEMENTATION AND ASSESSMENT				
6. Ensures ventilatory activity, checks airway				
7. Connects volumeter to airway				
8. Reassures patient				
9. Measures minute ventilation/observes response				
10. Restores patient to prior status				
11. Explains, demonstrates forced vital capacity maneuver				
12. Connects volumeter to airway				
13. Encourages/elicits maximum inspiration/forced expiration				
14. Repeats procedure for best patient effort				
15. Restores patient to prior status; reassures patient				
16. Explains, demonstrates inspiratory force maneuver				
17. Connect manometer/valve assembly to airway				
18. Blocks inspiratory gas flow, encourages maximum inspiration				
19. Repeats procedure for best patient effort				
20. Reassures patient; restores to prior status				
21. Calculates and interprets test results				
FOLLOW-UP				
22. Maintains/processes equipment				
23. Records pertinent data in chart and departmental records				
24. Notifies appropriate personnel				

STUDENT'S COMPREHENSION OF PROCEDURE (SELECT ONE ONLY)

The student demonstrates comprehensive knowledge of basic and advanced concepts beyond requirements of procedure	
The student demonstrates above average understanding of basic concepts applicable to the skill demonstrated	
The student demonstrates adequate knowledge of the essential elements of the task performed	
The student shows limited understanding of essential concepts related to the procedure	
The student has inadequate knowledge of even the basic concepts related to the task at hand	

OUTCOME CRITERIA (WHERE APPLICABLE)

☐ MET	SPECIFY CRITERIA NOT MET AND/OR PERTINENT CONSTRAINTS
☐ NOT MET	
☐ NOT APPL.	

ADDITIONAL COMMENTS

Include errors of omission or commission; if clinical therapeutic procedure emphasize communicative skills (verbal and non-verbal) and effectiveness of patient interaction:

SUMMARY PERFORMANCE EVALUATION AND RECOMMENDATIONS

SETTING	SATISFACTORY	UNSATISFACTORY	SPECIFY DEFICIENCIES
LABORATORY	☐ Can now perform skill under direct clinical supervision	☐ Requires additional laboratory practice	
CLINIC	☐ Ready for minimally supervised application and refinement	☐ Requires additional supervised clinical practice ☐ Complete re-evaluation required ☐ Re-evaluation·minor deficiencies only	

STUDENT: EVALUATOR: FACULTY:

PROCEDURAL SPECIFICATIONS
BEDSIDE VENTILATORY ASSESSMENT

I. Key Performance Elements

Procedural Element (Step)	Description of Satisfactory Performance
6. Ensures ventilatory activity, checks airway	Checks for spontaneously initiated respirations Stimulates/elicits spontaneous respirations Ensures patent/leak free airway
7. Connects volumeter to airway	Selects non-rebreathing valve if multiple patient use of volumeter Ensures device in off/reset position

9. Measures minute ventilation/ observes response	Initiates timed interval
	Observes patient for subjective signs of discomfort
	Observes changes in heart rate or rhythm
	Discontinues procedure if:
	  a. untoward changes in patient status
	  b. marked changes in cardiac rate/ rhythm
	Terminates timed interval
	Assesses validity of results

13. Encourages/elicits maximum inspiration/forced expiration	Ensures maximum inspiration Turns volumeter on at peak inspiration Verbally coaches full and forced expiration Observes patient for adverse response Modifies technique as necessary

18. Blocks inspiratory gas flow, encourages maximum inspiration

Blocks inspiratory gas flow for maximum of 20 seconds
Observes patient for subjective signs of discomfort
Observes changes in cardiac rate/rhythm
Discontinues procedure if:
a. untoward changes in patient status
b. marked changes in cardiac rate/rhythm
Assesses validity of results

20. Reassures patient; restores to prior status

Rechecks (readjusts) all parameters/alarm functions if patient on ventilator
Checks patient status (airway)
Reassures patient

II. Setting

The student is expected to demonstrate proficiency in bedside ventilatory assessment procedures in the following settings: (check those that apply)

☐ Laboratory   ☐ Other (specify)

☐ Clinic

_____

_____

III. Conditions

The student is expected to demonstrate proficiency in bedside ventilatory assessment procedures under the following conditions: (check those that apply)

Patient Variables

☐ Simulated (peer)

☐ Spontaneous breathing patient, normal airway
☐ Spontaneous breathing patient, artificial airway
☐ Patient receiving mechanical ventilation via artifical airway

Procedural Variables

☐ Minute ventilation

☐ Forced vital capacity

☐ Inspiratory force

Other conditional specifications: _____

_____

_____

IV. Equipment

The student is expected to demonstrate proficiency in bedside ventilatory assessment procedures using the following equipment: (check those that apply)

Airway Apparatus   Volumeter

☐ Mouthpiece   ☐ Mechanical turbine

☐ Mask   ☐ Electronic turbine

☐ Nonrebreathing   ☐ Electronic pneumotach
   valve   or flow tube

Other equipment specifications: _____

_____

_____

V. Outcome Criteria

The obtained measures of ventilatory function must correspond to those concurrently determined by the evaluator (degree of accuracy ± 5%).

VI. Oral Review Questions

1. What are the ranges of the measured parameters associated with:
   a. normal individuals?
   b. patients with ventilatory insufficiency?
   c. patients in ventilatory failure requiring mechanical ventilatory support?

2. What hazards, contraindications and precautions apply to the measurement procedures employed?

3. What are the sources of error encountered in making these bedside ventilatory measurements? How can such errors be minimized?

4. Interpret the physiological significance and potential cause(s) of the following observations made during bedside ventilatory assessment procedures:

   a. a 150 pound patient exhibits a minute ventilation of 20 liters/minute, at a frequency of 25/minute. Simultaneous measurement of the arterial partial pressure of carbon dioxide reveals a tension of 40 mmHg.

   b. during an inspiratory force maneuver, a monitored patient exhibits a drop in cardiac rate from 110 per minute to 38 per minute.

   c. prior to the measurement of minute ventilation, a patient receiving mechanical ventilatory support exhibits a pH of 7.52 with an arterial carbon dioxide tension of 29 mmHg. Upon initiation of the procedure, the patient remains apneic.

STUDENT:	DATE:

PROCEDURE (TASK): FORCED EXPIRATORY VOLUME

	SATISFACTORY	UNSATISFACTORY	NOT OBSERVED	NOT APPLICABLE
SETTING: ☐ LABORATORY ☐ OTHER: (SPECIFY) ☐ CLINIC				
CONDITIONS (DESCRIBE)				
EQUIPMENT UTILIZED:				

STEPS IN PROCEDURE OR TASK:

	SATISFACTORY	UNSATISFACTORY	NOT OBSERVED	NOT APPLICABLE
EQUIPMENT AND PATIENT PREPARATION	░	░	░	░
1. Verifies, interprets, and evaluates physician's orders				
2. Selects, gathers, and assembles appropriate equipment				
3. Confirms the functional operation (calibrates) the measurement system				
4. Identifies patient, self, and department				
5. Obtains/assesses pertinent pulmonary history, physical findings, applicable laboratory data (enters appropriate data)				
6. Explains procedure and confirms patient understanding				
IMPLEMENTATION AND ASSESSMENT	░	░	░	░
7. Connects patient to valve assembly (normal breathing)				
8. Initiates valve function				
9. Has patient take full inspiration/coordinates changeover				
10. Elicits forced/full expiration to residual volume (RV)				
11. Reassures patient				
12. Assesses test outcomes for reliability/validity				
13. Repeat procedure for best results/checks repeatibility				
14. Performs inspiratory capacity (IC), expiratory reserve volume (ERV)				
15. Performs maximum voluntary ventilation maneuver (MVV)				
16. Administers bronchodilator/waits for effect				
17. Repeats applicable procedures				
18. Calculates (obtains) patient, predicted, percent predicted values				
FOLLOW-UP	░	░	░	░
19. Maintains/processes equipment				
20. Records pertinent data in chart and departmental records				
21. Notifies appropriate personnel				

STUDENT'S COMPREHENSION OF PROCEDURE (SELECT ONE ONLY)

The student demonstrates comprehensive knowledge of basic and advanced concepts beyond requirements of procedure	
The student demonstrates above average understanding of basic concepts applicable to the skill demonstrated	
The student demonstrates adequate knowledge of the essential elements of the task performed	
The student shows limited understanding of essential concepts related to the procedure	
The student has inadequate knowledge of even the basic concepts related to the task at hand	

OUTCOME CRITERIA (WHERE APPLICABLE)

☐ MET	SPECIFY CRITERIA NOT MET AND/OR PERTINENT CONSTRAINTS
☐ NOT MET	
☐ NOT APPL.	

ADDITIONAL COMMENTS

Include errors of omission or commission; if clinical therapeutic procedure emphasize communicative skills (verbal and non-verbal) and effectiveness of patient interaction:

SUMMARY PERFORMANCE EVALUATION AND RECOMMENDATIONS

SETTING	SATISFACTORY	UNSATISFACTORY	SPECIFY DEFICIENCIES
LABORATORY	☐ Can now perform skill under direct clinical super-vision	☐ Requires additional laboratory practice	
CLINIC	☐ Ready for min-imally supervised application and refinement	☐ Requires additional supervised clinical practice ☐ Complete re-evaluation required ☐ Re-evaluation·minor deficiencies only	

STUDENT:　　　　　EVALUATOR:　　　　FACULTY:

PROCEDURAL SPECIFICATIONS
FORCED EXPIRATORY VOLUME

I. Key Performance Elements

Procedural Element (Step)	Description of Satisfactory Performance
3. Confirms the functional operation (calibrates) the measurement system	Checks circuit integrity Ensures proper valve function Checks (calibrates) volume/flow response of measurement apparatus Calibrates applicable gas analyzers
5. Obtains/assesses pertinent pulmonary history, physical findings, applicable laboratory data (enters appropriate data)	Elicits/records patient's pulmonary history Gather applicable laboratory data from chart/records Reviews (performs) physical assessment of thorax Refer to proficiency evaluation: PATIENT ASSESSMENT (Enters necessary data into computer)
12. Assesses test outcome for reliability/validity	Judges (where applicable) appropriateness of patient effort Inspects graphic results for artifact or evidence of inconsistencies Determines repeatability of results Indicates invalid or unreliable findings
14. Performs inspiratory capacity (IC), expiratory reserve volume (ERV)	Reassures patient Elicits maximum inspiration from functional residual capacity Has patient relax Elicits maximum expiration from functional residual capacity Repeats maneuvers if necessary

15. Performs maximum voluntary ventilation maneuver (MVV)

Reassures patient

Elicits maximum breathing effort (rate/depth)

Coaches patient to maintain rate/depth for designated interval

Terminates procedure, re-assures patient

II. Setting

The student is expected to demonstrate proficiency in the measurement of forced expiratory volume (and related procedures) in the following settings: (check those that apply)

☐ Laboratory

☐ Other (specify)

☐ Clinic

_____

_____

III. Conditions

The student is expected to demonstrate proficiency in the measurement of forced expiratory volume (and related procedures) under the following conditions: (check those that apply)

Patient Variables

☐ Simulated (peer)

☐ Known abnormalities, obstructive disease
☐ Known abnormalities, restrictive disease
☐ Unknown abnormalities

Procedure Variables

☐ Forced vital capacity only

☐ Maximum expiratory flow/ volume curve
☐ Maximum voluntary ventilation
☐ Pre/post assessment with bronchodilator

Other conditional specifications: _____

_____

_____

IV. Equipment

The student is expected to demonstrate proficiency in the measurement of forced expiratory volume (and related procedures) using the following equipment: (check those that apply)

Spirometer Type

☐ Water-sealed bell

☐ Rolling piston/bellows

☐ Wedge-type spirometer

☐ Electronic pneumotach

Recording Device

☐ Kymograph

☐ Strip chart recorder
   (volume vs. time)
☐ X-Y recorder
   (flow vs. volume)

System Variables

☐ Manual

☐ Computerized

Other equipment specifications: _____

_____

_____

V. Outcome Criteria

Measured parameters must be confirmed as repeatable by evaluator. Calculated values must correspond to those concurrently determined by evaluator (degree of accuracy ± 5%).

VI. Oral Review Questions

1. Draw, label, and differentiate between the components of the forced vital capacity curves (volume vs. time) characteristic of:
   a. normal pulmonary function
   b. restrictive lung disease
   c. chronic small airways obstruction

2. Draw, label, and differentiate between the components of maximum inspiratory/expiratory flow-volume curves characteristic of:
   a. fixed upper airway obstruction
   b. chronic obstructive (small airways) disease
   c. variable intrathoracic upper airway obstruction
   d. restrictive lung disease
   e. normal pulmonary function

3. Describe the physical principle and physiological significance of the volume of isoflow measurement.

4. Given three completed forced vital capacity maneuvers on three separate patients, properly interpret the results.

STUDENT:	DATE:				

PROCEDURE (TASK): FUNCTIONAL RESIDUAL CAPACITY					

	SATISFACTORY	UNSATISFACTORY	NOT OBSERVED	NOT APPLICABLE
SETTING: ☐ LABORATORY ☐ OTHER: (SPECIFY) ☐ CLINIC				
CONDITIONS (DESCRIBE)				
EQUIPMENT UTILIZED:				

STEPS IN PROCEDURE OR TASK:				
EQUIPMENT AND PATIENT PREPARATION	▨	▨	▨	▨
1. Verifies, interprets, and evaluates physician's orders				
2. Selects, gathers, and assembles appropriate equipment				
3. Confirms the functional operation (calibrates) the measurement system				
4. Identifies patient, self, and department				
5. Obtains/assesses pertinent pulmonary history, physical findings applicable laboratory data (enters appropriate data)				
6. Explains procedure and confirms patient understanding				
IMPLEMENTATION AND ASSESSMENT	▨	▨	▨	▨
7. Adds gas mixture to bell/reservoir; reads value(s)				
8. Connects patient to valve assembly				
9. Open valve at functional residual capacity/provides oxygen flow				
10. Elicits normal breathing by patient				
11. Checks gas concentrations at determined intervals				
12. Reassures patient				
13. Proceeds with test until equilibration; reads value(s)				
14. Restores patient to normal breathing				
15. Assesses test outcome for reliability/validity				
16. Calculates (obtains) patient, predicted, percent predicted values for appropriate volumes/capacities				
FOLLOW-UP	▨	▨	▨	▨
17. Maintains/processes equipment				
18. Records pertinent data in chart and department records				
19. Notifies appropriate personnel				

STUDENT'S COMPREHENSION OF PROCEDURE (SELECT ONE ONLY)

The student demonstrates comprehensive knowledge of basic and advanced concepts beyond requirements of procedure	
The student demonstrates above average understanding of basic concepts applicable to the skill demonstrated	
The student demonstrates adequate knowledge of the essential elements of the task performed	
The student shows limited understanding of essential concepts related to the procedure	
The student has inadequate knowledge of even the basic concepts related to the task at hand	

OUTCOME CRITERIA (WHERE APPLICABLE)

☐ MET	SPECIFY CRITERIA NOT MET AND/OR PERTINENT CONSTRAINTS
☐ NOT MET	
☐ NOT APPL.	

ADDITIONAL COMMENTS

Include errors of omission or commission; if clinical therapeutic procedure emphasize communicative skills (verbal and non-verbal) and effectiveness of patient interaction:

SUMMARY PERFORMANCE EVALUATION AND RECOMMENDATIONS

SETTING	SATISFACTORY	UNSATISFACTORY	SPECIFY DEFICIENCIES
LABORATORY	☐ Can now perform skill under direct clinical supervision	☐ Requires additional laboratory practice	
CLINIC	☐ Ready for minimally supervised application and refinement	☐ Requires additional supervised clinical practice ☐ Complete re-evaluation required ☐ Re-evaluation·minor deficiencies only	

STUDENT: EVALUATOR: FACULTY:

236

PROCEDURAL SPECIFICATIONS
FUNCTIONAL RESIDUAL CAPACITY

I. Key Performance Elements

Procedural Element (Step)	Description of Satisfactory Performance
3. Confirms the functional operation (calibrates) the measurement system	Checks circuit integrity Ensures proper valve function Checks (calibrates) volume/flow response of measurement apparatus Calibrates applicable gas analyzers
5. Obtains/assesses pertinent pulmonary history, physical findings, applicable laboratory data (enters appropriate data)	Elicits/records patient's pulmonary history Gather applicable laboratory data from chart/records Reviews (performs) physical assessment of thorax Refer to proficiency evaluation: PATIENT ASSESSMENT (Enters necessary data into computer)
15. Assesses test outcome for reliability/validity	Judges (where applicable) appropriateness of patient effort Inspects graphic results for artifacts or evidence of inconsistencies Determines repeatability of results Indicates invalid or unreliable findings

II. Setting

The student is expected to demonstrate proficiency in the measurement of functional residual capacity (and related volumes) in the following settings: (check those that apply)

☐ Laboratory   ☐ Other

☐ Clinic

_____

_____

III. Conditions

The student is expected to demonstrate proficiency in the measurement of functional residual capacity (and related volumes) under the following conditions: (check those that apply)

Patient Variables   Procedure Variables

☐ Simulated (peer)   ☐ Helium dilution

☐ Known abnormalities,   ☐ Nitrogen washout
   restrictive disease
☐ Known abnormalities,
   obstructive disease
☐ Unknown abnormalities

Other conditional specifications: _____

_____

_____

IV. Equipment

The equipment utilized for determination of functional residual capacity is dependent upon the procedural method employed (helium dilution or nitrogen washout) and is specified below

Equipment specification: _____

_____

_____

V. Outcome Criteria

Measured parameters must be confirmed as repeatable by the evaluator. Calculated values must coincide with those concurrently determined by the evaluator (degree of accuracy ± 5%).

VI. Oral Review Questions

1. Draw and label a graph which differentiates between all lung volumes and capacities. For each lung volume and capacity, specify the expected normal value (or range) for a 150 pound healthy male adult.

2. Differentiate between the necessary equipment, procedure, advantages and disadvantages of functional residual capacity determination by helium dilution versus nitrogen washout.

3. Differentiate between the "typical" alterations in lung volumes and capacities observed in restrictive and obstructive lung disease.

4. Describe the principle of measurement of lung volumes and capacities by body plethysmography. Explain why thoracic gas volumes measured by this method may often exceed those determined by gas equilibration techniques.

STUDENT:		DATE:				

PROCEDURE (TASK): DIFFUSING CAPACITY

	SATISFACTORY	UNSATISFACTORY	NOT OBSERVED	NOT APPLICABLE
SETTING: ☐ LABORATORY ☐ OTHER: (SPECIFY) ☐ CLINIC				
CONDITIONS (DESCRIBE)				
EQUIPMENT UTILIZED:				

STEPS IN PROCEDURE OR TASK:

	SATISFACTORY	UNSATISFACTORY	NOT OBSERVED	NOT APPLICABLE
EQUIPMENT AND PATIENT PREPARATION				
1. Verifies, interprets, and evaluates physician's order				
2. Selects, gathers, and assembles appropriate equipment				
3. Confirms the functional operation (calibrates) the measurement system				
4. Identifies patient, self, and department				
5. Obtains/assesses pertinent pulmonary history, physical findings, applicable laboratory data (enters appropriate data)				
6. Explains procedure and confirms patient understanding				
IMPLEMENTATION AND ASSESSMENT				
7. Fills carbon monoxide reservoir				
8. Connects patient to valve assembly				
9. Has patient exhale fully				
10. Initiates valve function				
11. Has patient take a full inspiration				
12. Ensures inspiratory hold for necessary time				
13. Collects sample during (slowed) patient exhalation				
14. Reads/records results; reassures patient				
15. Assesses test outcome for reliability/validity				
16. Repeat procedure if necessary				
17. Calculates test results				
FOLLOW-UP				
18. Maintains/processes equipment				
19. Records pertinent data in chart and department records				
20. Notifies appropriate personnel				

STUDENT'S COMPREHENSION OF PROCEDURE (SELECT ONE ONLY)

The student demonstrates comprehensive knowledge of basic and advanced concepts beyond requirements of procedure	
The student demonstrates above average understanding of basic concepts applicable to the skill demonstrated	
The student demonstrates adequate knowledge of the essential elements of the task performed	
The student shows limited understanding of essential concepts related to the procedure	
The student has inadequate knowledge of even the basic concepts related to the task at hand	

OUTCOME CRITERIA (WHERE APPLICABLE)

☐ MET	SPECIFY CRITERIA NOT MET AND/OR PERTINENT CONSTRAINTS
☐ NOT MET	
☐ NOT APPL.	

ADDITIONAL COMMENTS

Include errors of omission or commission; if clinical therapeutic procedure emphasize communicative skills (verbal and non-verbal) and effectiveness of patient interaction:

SUMMARY PERFORMANCE EVALUATION AND RECOMMENDATIONS

SETTING	SATISFACTORY	UNSATISFACTORY	SPECIFY DEFICIENCIES
LABORATORY	☐ Can now perform skill under direct clinical super- vision	☐ Requires additional laboratory practice	
CLINIC	☐ Ready for min- imally supervised application and refinement	☐ Requires additional supervised clinical practice ☐ Complete re- evaluation required ☐ Re-evaluation·minor deficiencies only	

STUDENT: EVALUATOR: FACULTY:

PROCEDURAL SPECIFICATIONS
DIFFUSING CAPACITY

I. Key Performance Elements

Procedural Element (Step)	Description of Satisfactory Performance
3. Confirms the functional operation (calibrates) the measurement system	Checks circuit integrity Ensures proper valve function Checks (calibrates volume/ flow response of measurement apparatus Calibrates applicable gas analyzers
5. Obtains/assesses pertinent pulmonary history, physical findings, applicable laboratory data (enters appropriate data)	Elicits/records patient's pulmonary history Gather applicable laboratory data from chart/records Reviews (performs) physical assessment of thorax Refer to proficiency evaluation: PATIENT ASSESSMENT (Enters necessary data into computer)
15. Assesses test outcome for reliability/validity	Judges (where applicable) appropriateness of patient effort Inspects graphic results for artifacts or evidence of inconsistencies Determines repeatability of results Indicates invalid or unreliable findings

II. Setting

The student is expected to demonstrate proficiency in the measurement of diffusing capacity in the following settings: (check those that apply)

☐ Laboratory

☐ Clinic

☐ Other (specify)

_____

_____

III. Conditions

The student is expected to demonstrate proficiency in the measurement of diffusing capacity under the following conditions: (check those that apply)

Patient Variables   Procedure Variables

☐ Simulated (peer)   ☐ Single-breath test

☐ Known abnormalities   ☐ Rebreathing technique

☐ Unknown abnormalities

Other conditional specifications: _____

_____

_____

IV. Equipment

The student is expected to demonstrate proficiency in the measurement of diffusing capacity with the following equipment: (check those that apply)

System Type   Automation

☐ Single-breath system   ☐ Manual

☐ Rebreathing system   ☐ Automated/computerized

Additional equipment specification: _____

_____

_____

V. Outcome Criteria

Measured parameters must be confirmed as repeatable by evaluator. Calculated values must correspond to those concurrently determined by the evaluator (degree of accuracy ± 5%)

VI. Oral Review Questions

1. Differentiate between the common anatomical/physiological processes causing a decrease in diffusing capacity of the lung.

2. Identify 2-3 causes for an increase in diffusing capacity of the lung.

3. Differentiate between the single breath and steady stage methods of determining diffusing capacity; state the normal values for each in proper units.

4. What is the rationale for the use of carbon monoxide as the test gas in diffusing capacity measurement? (Hint: be sure to differentiate between diffusion vs. perfusion limitations to gas transport across the alveolarcapillary membrane.)

STUDENT:	DATE:

PROCEDURE (TASK): ARTERIAL BLOOD GAS SAMPLING

SETTING: ☐ LABORATORY ☐ OTHER: (SPECIFY)
          ☐ CLINIC

CONDITIONS (DESCRIBE)

EQUIPMENT UTILIZED:

STEPS IN PROCEDURE OR TASK:	SATISFACTORY	UNSATISFACTORY	NOT OBSERVED	NOT APPLICABLE
EQUIPMENT AND PATIENT PREPARATION				
1. Washes hands				
2. Selects, gathers, and assembles appropriate equipment				
3. Verifies, interprets, and evaluates physician's order				
4. Checks chart for pertinent hematological information and compatibility of disease and procedure				
5. Identifies patient, self, and department				
6. Explains procedure and confirms patient understanding				
IMPLEMENTATION				
7. Tests for collateral circulation (Allen test)				
8. Prepares puncture site				
9. Prepares syringe (heparin)				
10. Palpates and anchors artery				
11. Reassures patient				
12. Penetrates artery, obtains sample				
13. Applies pressure to puncture site				
14. Caps syringe, ices sample				
15. Labels sample				
16. Reinspects puncture site				
17. Assures transportation and analysis of sample				
FOLLOW-UP				
18. Maintains/processes equipment				
19. Records pertinent data in chart and departmental records				
20. Notifies appropriate personnel				

STUDENT'S COMPREHENSION OF PROCEDURE (SELECT ONE ONLY)

The student demonstrates comprehensive knowledge of basic and advanced concepts beyond requirements of procedure	
The student demonstrates above average understanding of basic concepts applicable to the skill demonstrated	
The student demonstrates adequate knowledge of the essential elements of the task performed	
The student shows limited understanding of essential concepts related to the procedure	
The student has inadequate knowledge of even the basic concepts related to the task at hand	

OUTCOME CRITERIA (WHERE APPLICABLE)

☐ MET	SPECIFY CRITERIA NOT MET AND/OR PERTINENT CONSTRAINTS
☐ NOT MET	
☐ NOT APPL.	

ADDITIONAL COMMENTS

Include errors of omission or commission; if clinical therapeutic procedure emphasize communicative skills (verbal and non-verbal) and effectiveness of patient interaction:

SUMMARY PERFORMANCE EVALUATION AND RECOMMENDATIONS

SETTING	SATISFACTORY	UNSATISFACTORY	SPECIFY DEFICIENCIES
LABORATORY	☐ Can now perform skill under direct clinical supervision	☐ Requires additional laboratory practice	

CLINIC	☐ Ready for minimally supervised application and refinement	☐ Requires additional supervised clinical practice
		  ☐ Complete re-evaluation required
		  ☐ Re-evaluation·minor deficiencies only	

STUDENT: EVALUATOR: FACULTY:

PROCEDURAL SPECIFICATIONS
ARTERIAL BLOOD GAS SAMPLING

I. Key Performance Elements

Procedural Element (Step)	Description of Satisfactory Performance
7. Tests for collateral circulation (Allen Test)	Applies pressure to radial and ulnar arteries Has patient form tight fist Has patient relax hand Releases pressure from ulnar artery Observes response Releases pressure from radial artery Modifies procedure for unconscious/uncooperative patient
8. Prepares puncture site	Cleanses area over puncture site with disinfectant swab
9. Prepares syringe (heparin)	Maintains asepsis Aspirates heparin solution into syringe Coats internal syringe surface/barrel Expels excess heparin from syringe
10. Palpates and anchors artery	Positions/stabilizes puncture site Palpates point of maximum impulse with fingertips Anchors artery between fingertips

12. Penetrates artery, obtains sample

Minimizes angle between needle and artery
Advances needle upstream with bevel up
Adjusts position of needle until blood pulsates into syringe
Gathers sufficient sample volume
Withdraws needle/maintains angle
Repeats step 8-12 if:
a. needle withdrawn without sample
b. sample not obtained

13. Applies pressure to puncture site

Uses sterile gauze pad or dressing
Applies pressure for 2-5 minutes
Confirms stoppage of bleeding
Adjusts pressure application as necessary

14. Caps syringe, ices sample

Removes air bubbles from sample
Expels excess air
Caps syringe with stopper
Places syringe in ice bath

15. Labels sample

Lists patient name, room/bed number
Specifies oxygen concentration, ventilatory status

16. Reinspects puncture site

Assures bleeding stoppage
Observes for clot formation, blood infiltration or extravasation
Notes any untoward response

II. Setting

The student is expected to demonstrate proficiency in arterial blood gas sampling in the following settings: (check those that apply)

☐ Laboratory

☐ Clinic

☐ Other (specify)

_____

_____

III. Conditions

The student is expected to demonstrate proficiency in arterial blood gas sampling under the following conditions: (check those that apply)

Patient Variables

☐ Simulated (puncture arm)
☐ Unconscious patient

☐ Conscious patient

Procedure Variables

☐ Radial puncture

☐ Brachial puncture

☐ Femoral puncture

☐ Arterial line

Other conditional specifications: _____

_____

_____

IV. Equipment

The student is expected to demonstrate proficiency in arterial blood gas sampling with the following equipment: (check those that apply)

☐ Nondisposable components, glass syringe

☐ Disposable kit, glass syringe

☐ Disposable kit, plastic syringe

Other equipment specifications: _____

_____

_____

V. Outcome Criteria

A sufficient volume of (confirmed) arterial blood should be obtained with minimum patient discomfort and without unnecessary repeat puncture(s). After appropriate compression, the sample site should be free of blood extravasation. The obtained sample should be free of air bubbles, properly labeled, iced, and transported immediately for analysis.

VI. Oral Review Questions

1. What hazards and complications are associated with arterial blood gas sampling via needle puncture? What are the clinical manifestations of these complications? How can these hazards and complications be minimized?

2. What effect will the following conditions have upon measured arterial blood gas parameters?
    a. warming of the sample?
    b. excess air in the syringe?
    c. excess heparin in the syringe?
    d. delay in the analysis of the sample?

3. Why is the radial artery generally preferred as the site for arterial blood gas sampling?

4. What effects do patient temperature variations have upon blood gas parameters measured at the standard 37° C? How can these variations be accounted for?

STUDENT:	DATE:				

PROCEDURE (TASK): ARTERIAL BLOOD GAS ANALYSIS

	SATISFACTORY	UNSATISFACTORY	NOT OBSERVED	NOT APPLICABLE
SETTING: ☐ LABORATORY ☐ OTHER: (SPECIFY) ☐ CLINIC				
CONDITIONS (DESCRIBE)				
EQUIPMENT UTILIZED:				

STEPS IN PROCEDURE OR TASK:

	SATISFACTORY	UNSATISFACTORY	NOT OBSERVED	NOT APPLICABLE
EQUIPMENT PREPARATION				
1. Activates analyzer, provides warm-up				
2. Inspects electrodes, analysis chamber				
3. Assures patency/function of fluid and gas lines				
4. Gathers necessary solutions and controls				
5. Calculates calibrating gas partial pressures (enters data)				
6. Balances/slopes pH and gas electrodes				
7. Confirms accuracy with control values				
IMPLEMENTATION				
8. Repeats balance calibration				
9. Mixes sample				
10. Introduces sample into analysis chamber				
11. Reads and records appropriate parameters				
12. Flushes analysis chamber				
FOLLOW-UP				
13. Calculates derived parameters				
14. Records results in departmental records				
15. Notifies appropriate personnel				
16. Maintains/processes equipment				

STUDENT'S COMPREHENSION OF PROCEDURE (SELECT ONE ONLY)

The student demonstrates comprehensive knowledge of basic and advanced concepts beyond requirements of procedure	
The student demonstrates above average understanding of basic concepts applicable to the skill demonstrated	
The student demonstrates adequate knowledge of the essential elements of the task performed	
The student shows limited understanding of essential concepts related to the procedure	
The student has inadequate knowledge of even the basic concepts related to the task at hand	

OUTCOME CRITERIA (WHERE APPLICABLE)

☐ MET	SPECIFY CRITERIA NOT MET AND/OR PERTINENT CONSTRAINTS
☐ NOT MET	
☐ NOT APPL.	

ADDITIONAL COMMENTS

Include errors of omission or commission; if clinical therapeutic procedure emphasize communicative skills (verbal and non-verbal) and effectiveness of patient interaction:

SUMMARY PERFORMANCE EVALUATION AND RECOMMENDATIONS

SETTING	SATISFACTORY	UNSATISFACTORY	SPECIFY DEFICIENCIES
LABORATORY	☐ Can now perform skill under direct clinical supervision	☐ Requires additional laboratory practice	
CLINIC	☐ Ready for minimally supervised application and refinement	☐ Requires additional supervised clinical practice ☐ Complete re-evaluation required ☐ Re-evaluation·minor deficiencies only	

STUDENT: EVALUATOR: FACULTY:

PROCEDURAL SPECIFICATIONS
ARTERIAL BLOOD GAS ANALYSIS

I. Key Performance Elements

Procedural Element (Step)	Description of Satisfactory Performance
5. Calculates calibrating gas partial pressures (enters data)	Determines barometric pressure Uses water vapor correction factor Calculates partial pressures in mmHg (Enters values into computer)
6. Balances/slopes pH and gas electrodes	Introduces high buffer Balances pH display to high buffer value Flushes analysis chamber Introduces low buffer Slopes pH display to low buffer value Flushes analysis chamber Introduces low calibrating gas Balances gas partial pressure displays to calculated value Introduces high calibrating gas Slopes gas partial pressure displays to calculated value (Confirms automated calibration)
7. Confirms accuracy with control values	Prepares control solutions Introduces controls into analysis chamber Reads/records control values Compares measured values to control ranges Repeats calibration/control tests until response within normal limits
9. Mixes sample	Removes visible air bubbles Expels excess heparin Rolls sample between palms of hands

13. Calculates derived parameters

Selects appropriate nomograms
Calculates derived values
Corrects for patient variables
Rechecks calculations for
accuracy

II. Setting

The student is expected to demonstrate proficiency in the
analysis of arterial blood gas samples in the following settings:
(check those that apply)

☐ Laboratory

☐ Clinic

☐ Other (specify)

_____

_____

III. Conditions

The student is expected to demonstrate proficiency in the
analysis of arterial blood gas samples under the following
conditions: (check those that apply)

Sample Variables

☐ Simulated (tonometered
blood or controls
only)
☐ Patient sample, unknown
values
☐ Patient sample, known
values

Procedure Variables

☐ Manual analysis

☐ Semi-automated analysis

☐ Fully-automated analysis

Other conditional specifications: _____

_____

_____

IV. Equipment

The student is expected to demonstrate proficiency in the analysis of arterial blood gas samples using the following equipment:
(check those that apply)

Analyzer Type

☐ Manual

Manufacturer/Model (specify)

_____

_____

☐ Semi-automated

_____

_____

☐ Fully-automated

_____

_____

Other equipment specifications: _____

_____

_____

V. Outcome Criteria

After calibration, analysis of control values should yield results
within normal limits of accuracy. Measured sample values, and
those derived by calculation(s) should coincide with those
concurrently determined by the evaluator (range of accuracy ±
5%).

VI. Oral Review Questions

1. Describe the theory and principle of operation of the pH,
   pCO_2 and pO_2 electrodes.

2. Differentiate between the principles of slope and balance of an
   electrical instrument and describe the effect of "drift" upon
   the reliability and accuracy of blood gas measurements.

3. What are the most common errors encountered in blood gas
   analysis? How can they be identified? How can they be
   rectified or eliminated?

4. Describe the necessary components of a quality assurance
   program for blood gas analysis.

5. Given five complete blood gas analysis reports, and pertinent
   patient information:
   a. assess the values for consistency
   b. determine the patient's acid-base status
   c. evaluate the adequacy of the patient's oxygenation
   d. identify the factor(s) contributing to any observed
      abnormalities in acid-base balance or oxygenation
   e. recommend, where indicated, appropriate therapeutic
      intervention.

VENTILATORY CARE

STUDENT:	DATE:				

PROCEDURE (TASK): VENTILATOR PREPARATION AND APPLICATION					

	SATISFACTORY	UNSATISFACTORY	NOT OBSERVED	NOT APPLICABLE
SETTING: ☐ LABORATORY ☐ OTHER: (SPECIFY) ☐ CLINIC				
CONDITIONS (DESCRIBE)				
EQUIPMENT UTILIZED:				

STEPS IN PROCEDURE OR TASK:

EQUIPMENT PREPARATION				
1. Washes hands				
2. Verifies, interprets, and evaluates physician's orders				
3. Selects, gathers, and assembles ventilator and circuitry				
4. Fills humidifier with sterile, distilled water				
5. Completes operational check of ventilator function				
6. Determines appropriate mode of ventilation				
7. Determines and sets appropriate ventilatory parameters				
8. Sets initial flowrate for proper inspiratory/expiratory rate				

PATIENT PREPARATION				
9. Identifies patient, self, and department				
10. Explains procedure and confirms patient understanding				

IMPLEMENTATION AND ASSESSMENT				
11. Attaches patient to ventilator during expiration				
12. Sets all alarm functions				
13. Confirms ventilator rate (patient spontaneous rate)				
14. Assesses patient response				
15. Draws or has drawn an arterial blood gas				
16. Readjusts parameters according to blood gas data				
17. Repeats steps 13 - 15 until patient stabilized				

FOLLOW-UP				
18. Maintains/processes equipment				
19. Records pertinent data in chart and departmental records				
20. Notifies appropriate personnel				

STUDENT'S COMPREHENSION OF PROCEDURE (SELECT ONE ONLY)

The student demonstrates comprehensive knowledge of basic and advanced concepts beyond requirements of procedure	
The student demonstrates above average understanding of basic concepts applicable to the skill demonstrated	
The student demonstrates adequate knowledge of the essential elements of the task performed	
The student shows limited understanding of essential concepts related to the procedure	
The student has inadequate knowledge of even the basic concepts related to the task at hand	

OUTCOME CRITERIA (WHERE APPLICABLE)

☐ MET	SPECIFY CRITERIA NOT MET AND/OR PERTINENT CONSTRAINTS
☐ NOT MET	
☐ NOT APPL.	

ADDITIONAL COMMENTS

Include errors of omission or commission; if clinical therapeutic procedure emphasize communicative skills (verbal and non-verbal) and effectiveness of patient interaction:

SUMMARY PERFORMANCE EVALUATION AND RECOMMENDATIONS

SETTING	SATISFACTORY	UNSATISFACTORY	SPECIFY DEFICIENCIES
LABORATORY	☐ Can now perform skill under direct clinical supervision	☐ Requires additional laboratory practice	

CLINIC	☐ Ready for minimally supervised application and refinement	☐ Requires additional supervised clinical practice
		  ☐ Complete re-evaluation required
		  ☐ Re-evaluation·minor deficiencies only	

STUDENT: EVALUATOR: FACULTY:

PROCEDURAL SPECIFICATIONS
VENTILATOR PREPARATION AND APPLICATION

I. Key Performance Elements

Procedural Element (Step)	Description of Satisfactory Performance
3. Selects, gathers, and assembles ventilator circuitry	Maintains asepsis Checks circuitry for leaks Measures/confirms circuit compliance factor
5. Completes operational check of ventilator function	Follows manufacturer's (or departmental) operating procedure Confirms function of all pertinent controls and alarms Confirms accuracy of all applicable parameters Troubleshoots functional abnormalities; replaces ventilator if not correctable
6. Determines appropriate mode of ventilation	Selects control, assist/control or intermittent ventilatory mode according to physician's order or appropriate clinical indications
7. Determines and sets appropriate ventilatory parameters	Utilizes body weight formula or equivalent to estimate tidal volume Selects frequency appropriate for mode Selects oxygen concentration as indicated by clinical circumstances Determines need for/selects appropriate end expiratory pressure level Refer to proficiency evaluations: IMV, WEANING AND VENTILATOR DISCONTINUOUS, and CONTINUOUS DISTENDING PRESSURE THERAPY

8. Sets initial flowrate for proper inspiratory/expiratory ratio	Sets flowrate as indicated by clinical circumstances Confirms preset inspiratory/ expiratory time ratio (control, assist/control)
12. Sets all alarm functions	Ensures disconnect indicator(s) operative Limits pressure at appropriate level Provides accessory alarm functions where indicated or necessary
14. Assesses patient response	Compares preset values with those obtained Adjust preset values accordingly Auscultates thorax for breath sounds Observes pattern of ventilation, signs of oxygenation Assesses (preliminary) cardiovascular response Refer to proficiency evaluations: VITAL SIGNS, BLOOD PRESSURE, and PATIENT ASSESSMENT
15. Draws or has drawn an arterial blood gas	Refer to proficiency evaluation: ARTERIAL BLOOD GAS SAMPLING
16. Readjusts parameters according to blood gas data	Adjusts tidal volume/minute ventilation to achieve (patient) normal pH Adjusts oxygen concentration/ distending pressure to ensure adequate oxygenation

II. Setting

The student is expected to demonstrate proficiency in the preparation and application of mechanical ventilators in the following settings: (check those that apply)

☐ Laboratory   ☐ Other (specify)

☐ Clinic

_____

_____

III. Conditions

The student is expected to demonstrate proficiency in the preparation and application of mechanical ventilators under the following conditions: (check those that apply)

Patient Variables   Procedure Variables

☐ Simulated (manikin   ☐ Control mode
   or lung analog)
☐ Neonate/Infant   ☐ Assist/control mode

☐ Child   ☐ Intermittent ventilatory
                              mode(s)
☐ Adult   ☐ In conjunction with
                              expiratory positive
                              pressure (PEEP)

Other conditional specifications: _____

_____

_____

IV. Equipment

The student is expected to demonstrate proficiency in the preparation and application of mechanical ventilators using the following equipment: (check those that apply)

Ventilator Type   Manufacturer/Model (specify)

☐ Adult volume or   _____
   time cycled
                             _____

                             _____

                             _____

                             _____

☐ Pediatric/Neonatal   _____
   volume or time
   cycled   _____

                             _____

                             _____

                             _____

☐ General duty
pressure cycled

_____

_____

_____

_____

Other equipment specifications: _____

_____

_____

V. Outcome Criteria

Prior to application, the functional operation of the ventilator
must be confirmed according to the manufacturer's (or
departmental) specifications. After application and (where
necessary) adjustment of appropriate parameters, the patient's
acid-base balance and oxygenation should be optimized, as
indicated or desired in the particular circumstances at hand.

VI. Oral Review Questions

1. For the specific equipment applied:
   a. classify the ventilator
   b. specify the range of available parameters, modes and
      functions applicable to the unmodified ventilator
   c. Describe how the ventilator controls the following:
      time parameters
      sensitivity
      delivered volume
      oxygen concentration
      sign volumes
      waveform modifications
      spontaneous breathing modes
   d. Describe the clinical indications, contraindications, and
      hazards of the mode of ventilation employed.

STUDENT:		DATE:				

PROCEDURE (TASK): ROUTINE VENTILATOR CHECK						

SETTING: ☐ LABORATORY ☐ OTHER: (SPECIFY) ☐ CLINIC	SATISFACTORY	UNSATISFACTORY	NOT OBSERVED	NOT APPLICABLE
CONDITIONS (DESCRIBE)				
EQUIPMENT UTILIZED:				

STEPS IN PROCEDURE OR TASK:				
EQUIPMENT AND PATIENT PREPARATION				
1. Washes hands				
2. Selects, gathers, and assembles appropriate equipment				
3. Verifies, interprets, and evaluates physician's order				
4. Identifies patient, self, and department				
5. Explains procedure and confirms patient understanding				
IMPLEMENTATION AND ASSESSMENT				
6. Verifies current ventilator settings				
7. Checks humidifier function and water level				
8. Refills humidifier				
9. Checks airway temperature				
10. Checks circuit integrity for leaks/obstructions and position				
11. Inspects and assesses patient status				
12. Correlates pre-set values with those monitored				
13. Ensures proper ventilator function (troubleshoots)				
14. Verifies all alarms functions/settings				
15. Reassures patient				
FOLLOW-UP				
16. Maintains/processes equipment				
17. Records pertinent data in chart and departmental records				
18. Notifies appropriate personnel				

STUDENT'S COMPREHENSION OF PROCEDURE (SELECT ONE ONLY)

The student demonstrates comprehensive knowledge of basic and advanced concepts beyond requirements of procedure	
The student demonstrates above average understanding of basic concepts applicable to the skill demonstrated	
The student demonstrates adequate knowledge of the essential elements of the task performed	
The student shows limited understanding of essential concepts related to the procedure	
The student has inadequate knowledge of even the basic concepts related to the task at hand	

OUTCOME CRITERIA (WHERE APPLICABLE)

☐ MET	SPECIFY CRITERIA NOT MET AND/OR PERTINENT CONSTRAINTS
☐ NOT MET	
☐ NOT APPL.	

ADDITIONAL COMMENTS

Include errors of omission or commission; if clinical therapeutic procedure emphasize communicative skills (verbal and non-verbal) and effectiveness of patient interaction:

SUMMARY PERFORMANCE EVALUATION AND RECOMMENDATIONS

SETTING	SATISFACTORY	UNSATISFACTORY	SPECIFY DEFICIENCIES
LABORATORY	☐ Can now perform skill under direct clinical supervision	☐ Requires additional laboratory practice	
CLINIC	☐ Ready for minimally supervised application and refinement	☐ Requires additional supervised clinical practice ☐ Complete re-evaluation required ☐ Re-evaluation·minor deficiencies only	

STUDENT: EVALUATOR: FACULTY:

PROCEDURAL SPECIFICATIONS
ROUTINE VENTILATOR CHECK

I. Key Performance Elements

Procedural Element (Step)	Description of Satisfactory Performance
6. Verifies current ventilator settings	Ensures correspondence between physician's orders and pre-set values Identifies discrepancies Readjusts discrepant values to correlate with physician's orders Contacts physician regarding discrepant values
8. Refills humidifier	Maintains asepsis Empties humidifier in wash sink Refills with sterile distilled water to indicated level Checks for proper seal/leaks
9. Checks airway temperature	Waits sufficient time after humidifier refill for warm-up Ensures airway temperature of 35-37° C Checks/confirms airway temperature controls/alarm functions
10. Checks circuit integrity for leaks/obstructions and position	Drains tubing away from patient into disposal Cycles ventilator against sterile obstruction, confirms pressure limiting Checks/minimizes traction on artificial airway (repositions circuit)
11. Inspects and assesses patient status	Refer to proficiency evaluations: VITAL SIGNS, BLOOD PRESSURE, PATIENT ASSESSMENT, CUFF MANAGEMENT, and TRACHEOBRONCHIAL ASPIRATION Records pertinent observations

12. Correlates pre-set values with those monitored

Measures expired tidal volumes, compares to pre-set value

Measures/records ventilator rate and patient spontaneous rate

Measures F_IO_2, compares to pre-set value

Accounts for discrepancies in values

13. Ensures proper ventilator function (troubleshoots)

Identifies discrepancies in parameters of ventilation/oxygenation

Differentiates between patient and mechanical problems

Solves problem or provides interim corrective measures

Disconnects ventilator/provides manual support if in doubt

17. Records pertinent data in chart and departmental records

Updates flowsheets

Confirms (by signature) all entries

Notes patient status

II. Setting

The student is expected to demonstrate proficiency in the routine check of patients receiving mechanical ventilation in the following settings: (check those that apply)

☐ Laboratory

☐ Clinic

☐ Other (specify)

_____

_____

III. Conditions

The student is expected to demonstrate proficiency in the routine check of patients receiving mechanical ventilation under the following conditions: (check those that apply)

Patient Variables

☐ Simulated (manikin or analog)

☐ Infant/neonate

☐ Child

☐ Adult

Procedure Variables

☐ Check only

☐ In conjunction with circuitry change

Other conditional specifications: _____

_____

_____

IV. Equipment

The student is expected to demonstrate proficiency in the routine check of patients receiving mechanical ventilation using the following equipment: (check those that apply)

Ventilator Type

☐ Adult volume or time cycled

☐ Pediatric/neonatal volume or time cycled

☐ General duty pressure cycled

Manufacturer/Model (specify)

_____

_____

_____

_____

_____

_____

_____

_____

_____

_____

_____

Other equipment specifications: _____

_____

_____

V. Outcome Criteria

Discrepancies between all established and observed parameters must be identified and, where possible, rectified. Circuit integrity must be confirmed. Any untoward patient response must be identified and, where indicated, appropriate corrective action must be taken. All records must be accurate and complete.

VI. Oral Review Questions

1. Identify the likely cause and appropriate action necessary when the following observations are noted on a routine ventilator check:
   Patient behaviors:
      a. restlessness, agitation
      b. confusion, disorientation
      c. somnolence, obtundation
      d. dyspnea
      e. headache
      f. twitching, tetany, convulsions
      g. asterixis
   Vital signs
      a. hypotension
      b. hypertension
      c. respiratory swings of blood pressure
      d. decreased urinary output
      e. weight gain
      f. changes in respiratory rate
   Chest signs
      a. asynchrony with the ventilator
      b. decreased breath sounds
      c. ronchi or wheezes
   Skin changes
      a. cool skin, diminished pulses
      b. hot moist skin
      c. crepitus
   Airway
      a. inspissated secretions
      b. inability to achieve cuff seal
   Ventilator changes
      a. increased maximum airway pressure
      b. I/E ratio excessively high
      c. increased minute volume (assist/control mode)
      d. changes in PEEP levels
      e. F_IO_2 drift

STUDENT:	DATE:				

PROCEDURE (TASK): IMV, WEANING, VENTILATOR DISCONTINUANCE

SETTING: ☐ LABORATORY ☐ OTHER: (SPECIFY) ☐ CLINIC	SATISFACTORY	UNSATISFACTORY	NOT OBSERVED	NOT APPLICABLE
CONDITIONS (DESCRIBE)				
EQUIPMENT UTILIZED:				

STEPS IN PROCEDURE OR TASK:

	SATISFACTORY	UNSATISFACTORY	NOT OBSERVED	NOT APPLICABLE
EQUIPMENT AND PATIENT PREPARATION	▨	▨	▨	▨
1. Washes hands				
2. Selects, gathers, and assembles appropriate equipment				
3. Verifies, interprets, and evaluates physician's order				
4. Identifies patient, self, and department				
5. Explains procedure and confirms patient understanding				
IMPLEMENTATION AND ASSESSMENT	▨	▨	▨	▨
6. Obtains baseline physiological profile				
7. Performs operational check of equipment function				
8. Reassures patient				
9. Initiates IMV mode (weaning procedure)				
10. Assesses patient's response				
11. Readjusts therapy as indicated (reassures patient)				
12. Monitors patient progress				
FOLLOW-UP	▨	▨	▨	▨
13. Provides appropriate follow-up care				
14. Records pertinent data in chart and departmental records				
15. Maintains/processes equipment				
16. Notifies appropriate personnel				

STUDENT'S COMPREHENSION OF PROCEDURE (SELECT ONE ONLY)

The student demonstrates comprehensive knowledge of basic and advanced concepts beyond requirements of procedure	
The student demonstrates above average understanding of basic concepts applicable to the skill demonstrated	
The student demonstrates adequate knowledge of the essential elements of the task performed	
The student shows limited understanding of essential concepts related to the procedure	
The student has inadequate knowledge of even the basic concepts related to the task at hand	

OUTCOME CRITERIA (WHERE APPLICABLE)

☐ MET	SPECIFY CRITERIA NOT MET AND/OR PERTINENT CONSTRAINTS
☐ NOT MET	
☐ NOT APPL.	

ADDITIONAL COMMENTS

Include errors of omission or commission; if clinical therapeutic procedure emphasize communicative skills (verbal and non-verbal) and effectiveness of patient interaction:

SUMMARY PERFORMANCE EVALUATION AND RECOMMENDATIONS

SETTING	SATISFACTORY	UNSATISFACTORY	SPECIFY DEFICIENCIES
LABORATORY	☐ Can now perform skill under direct clinical supervision	☐ Requires additional laboratory practice	
CLINIC	☐ Ready for minimally supervised application and refinement	☐ Requires additional supervised clinical practice ☐ Complete re-evaluation required ☐ Re-evaluation·minor deficiencies only	

STUDENT: EVALUATOR: FACULTY:

PROCEDURAL SPECIFICATIONS
IMV, WEANING AND VENTILATOR DISCONTINUANCE

I. Key Performance Elements

Procedural Element (Step)	Description of Satisfactory Performance
6. Obtains baseline physiological profile	Collects/calculates (where available) pertinent data on adequacy of oxygenation, ventilation, mechanics and cardiovascular performance, to include a. PaO_2, $P(A-a)O_2$, shunt fraction b. Blood pressure, cardiac rate, rhythm, cardiac output/index c. $\dot{V}E$, FVC, IF d. $PaCO_2$, VD/VT
7. Performs operational check of equipment function	Checks patency of delivery system Checks operation of accessory equipment (blenders/ humidifiers, etc.) Ensures operation of relief valves, venturi systems, reservoirs, and breathing valves Confirms alarm/indicator and safety systems Replaces defective or inoperable equipment/components
9. Initiates, IMV mode (weaning procedure)	Opens patient to IMV circuit Lowers ventilator rate Coaches patient with spontaneous breathing Adjusts appropriate indicator/ alarm systems 　　　OR Removes patient from ventilator Provides appropriate weaning therapy Coaches patient with spontaneous breathing

10. Assesses patient's response	Repeats (at appropriate intervals) collection/ calculation of physiological data (#6 above) and subjective observations of patient comfort, fatigue, etc.
11. Readjusts therapy as indi- cated (reassures patient)	Restores patient to full ventilatory support if: a. marked deterioration in physiological para- meters b. evidence of severe physical discomfort or psychological stress
12. Monitors patient progress	Repeats (at appropriate intervals) collection/ calculation of physio- logical data (#6 above) and subjective obser- vations of patient comfort, fatigue, etc., until stable and acceptable conditions are achieved
13. Provides appropriate follow-up care	Maintains adequate humidifi- cation Ensures appropriate oxygen- ation Maintains airway patency Refer to proficiency evalua- tions: OXYGEN THERAPY, AEROSOL/HUMIDITY THERAPY, TRACHEO- BRONCHIAL ASPIRATION, and ENDOTRACHEAL EXTUBATION

II. Setting

The student is expected to demonstrate proficiency in the application of IMV, weaning, and ventilator discontinuance procedures in the following settings: (check those that apply)

☐ Laboratory

☐ Clinic

☐ Other (specify)

_____

_____

III. Conditions

The student is expected to demonstrate proficiency in the application of IMV, weaning, and ventilator discontinuance procedures under the following conditions: (check those that apply)

Patient Variables

☐ Simulated (manikin or analog)
☐ Infant/neonate

☐ Child

☐ Adult

Procedure Variables

☐ IMV as primary ventilatory mode
☐ IMV applied for weaning

☐ Alternative weaning procedure

Other conditional specifications: _____

_____

_____

IV. Equipment

The student is expected to demonstrate proficiency in the application of IMV, weaning, and ventilator discontinuance procedures using the following equipment: (check those that apply)

IMV System Type

☐ Continuous flow IMV

   ☐ Ambient reservoir

   ☐ Pressure reservoir

☐ Demand flow IMV

   ☐ Mandatory

   ☐ Synchronous

Manufacturer/Specifications

_____

_____

_____

_____

_____

_____

_____

_____

Other equipment specifications: _____

_____

_____

IV. Equipment

Additional equipment (where required) includes that applicable to the proficiency evaluations: BEDSIDE VENTILATORY ASSESSMENT, ARTERIAL BLOOD GAS SAMPLING, ARTERIAL BLOOD GAS ANALYSIS, OXYGEN THERAPY, AEROSOL/HUMIDITY THERAPY, TRACHEOBRONCHIAL ASPIRATION, and ENDOTRACHEAL EXTUBATION.

V. Outcome Criteria

The goals of instituting the IMV, weaning, or ventilator discontinuance procedure, where possible, should be achieved without untoward patient response.

VI. Oral Review Questions

1. What are the clinical indications, desirable and undesirable physiological effects, hazards and contraindications to the utilization of IMV/SIMV techniques?

2. Differentiate between the principles of operation, advantages, disadvantages, capabilities, and limitations of the following types of IMV systems:
   Continuous flow IMV
      a. ambient reservoir modifications
      b. pressure reservoir modifications
   Demand flow IMV
      a. mandatory, nonsynchronized
      b. synchronized (SIMV)

3. Specify the physiological criteria necessary for consideration of ventilator discontinuance in adult patients receiving mechanical ventilatory support.

STUDENT:	DATE:

PROCEDURE (TASK): CONTINUOUS DISTENDING PRESSURE THERAPY

SETTING: ☐ LABORATORY ☐ OTHER: (SPECIFY)
 ☐ CLINIC

CONDITIONS (DESCRIBE)

EQUIPMENT UTILIZED:

STEPS IN PROCEDURE OR TASK:	SATISFACTORY	UNSATISFACTORY	NOT OBSERVED	NOT APPLICABLE
EQUIPMENT AND PATIENT PREPARATION	▨	▨	▨	▨
1. Washes hands				
2. Selects, gathers, and assembles appropriate equipment				
3. Verifies, interprets, and evaluates physician's order				
4. Identifies patient, self, and department				
5. Explains procedure and confirms patient's understanding				
IMPLEMENTATION AND ASSESSMENT	▨	▨	▨	▨
6. Obtains baseline physiological profile				
7. Performs operational check of equipment function				
8. Reassures patient				
9. Initiates continuous distending pressure				
10. Ensures appropriate pressure level				
11. Assesses patient's response				
12. Readjusts pressure to optimal level (reassures patient)				
13. Monitors patient progress				
FOLLOW-UP	▨	▨	▨	▨
14. Provides appropriate follow-up care/monitoring				
15. Records pertinent data in chart and departmental records				
16. Maintains/processes equipment				
17. Notifies appropriate personnel				

STUDENT'S COMPREHENSION OF PROCEDURE (SELECT ONE ONLY)

The student demonstrates comprehensive knowledge of basic and advanced concepts beyond requirements of procedure	
The student demonstrates above average understanding of basic concepts applicable to the skill demonstrated	
The student demonstrates adequate knowledge of the essential elements of the task performed	
The student shows limited understanding of essential concepts related to the procedure	
The student has inadequate knowledge of even the basic concepts related to the task at hand	

OUTCOME CRITERIA (WHERE APPLICABLE)

☐ MET	SPECIFY CRITERIA NOT MET AND/OR PERTINENT CONSTRAINTS
☐ NOT MET	
☐ NOT APPL.	

ADDITIONAL COMMENTS

Include errors of omission or commission; if clinical therapeutic procedure emphasize communicative skills (verbal and non-verbal) and effectiveness of patient interaction:

SUMMARY PERFORMANCE EVALUATION AND RECOMMENDATIONS

SETTING	SATISFACTORY	UNSATISFACTORY	SPECIFY DEFICIENCIES
LABORATORY	☐ Can now perform skill under direct clinical supervision	☐ Requires additional laboratory practice	
CLINIC	☐ Ready for minimally supervised application and refinement	☐ Requires additional supervised clinical practice ☐ Complete re-evaluation required ☐ Re-evaluation·minor deficiencies only	

STUDENT: EVALUATOR: FACULTY:

280

PROCEDURAL SPECIFICATIONS
CONTINUOUS DISTENDING PRESSURE THERAPY

I. Key Performance Elements

Procedural Element (Step)	Description of Satisfactory Performance
6. Obtains baseline physiological profile	Collects/calculates (where available) pertinent data on adequacy of oxygenation and cardiovascular performance, to include: a. PaO_2. $P(A-a)O_2$, shunt fraction b. blood pressure, cardiac rate, rhythm, cardiac output/index c. pulmonary vascular resistance d. lung/thorax compliance
7. Performs operational check of equipment function	Connects system to test lung or analog Adjusts pressure to level specified Checks system for leaks Adjusts flow or sensitivity Confirms sensitivity (if demand valve) Confirms pressure level Confirms safety relief function Confirms disconnect or low pressure alarm indicator
10. Ensures appropriate pressure level	Adjusts flow in continuous flow systems to 2–3 patient's minute ventilation Confirms ventilator cycling/demand valve function by observing manometer/spontaneous breath indicators Adjusts flow or sensitivity to minimize work, maintain appropriate pressure level Adjusts low pressure alarm to level below pressure selected

	Adjust volumetric alarm to volume less than minimum desirable spontaneous volume of patient
11. Assess patient's response	Observes patient for subjective signs of discomfort, anxiety Observes changes in subjective signs of hypoxemia or hypercapnea Determines (subjectively) changes in the work of breathing (accessory muscle use/retractions, rate of breathing, etc.) Observes changes in heart rate or rhythm Measures blood pressure, notes changes from baseline Auscultates thorax Repeats step #6 Notes/interprets changes from baseline measurements
12. Readjusts distending pressure to optimum level (reassures patient)	Provides for satisfactory oxygenation without cardiovascular depression and a minimal likelihood of oxygen toxicity
13. Monitors patient progress	Follows oxygenation status by collection/recording of appropriate objective data Follows maintenance of adequate perfusion by collection/recording of appropriate objective data Makes recommendations on level/continuance of therapy based upon patient status/progress

II. Setting

The student is expected to demonstrate proficiency in the application of continuous distending pressure therapy in the following settings: (check those that apply)

☐ Laboratory   ☐ Other (specify)

☐ Clinic

_____

_____

III. Conditions

The student is expected to demonstrate proficiency in the application of continuous distending pressure therapy under the following conditions: (check those that apply)

Patient Variables   Procedure Variables

☐ Simulated (manikin   ☐ In conjunction with me-
   or analog)   chanical ventilation (PEEP)
☐ Infant/neonate   ☐ Without mechanical
                               ventilatory sup-
☐ Child   port (CPAP)

☐ Adult

Other conditional specifications: _____

_____

_____

IV. Equipment

The student is expected to demonstrate proficiency in the application of continuous distending pressure therapy using the following equipment: (check those that apply)

Equipment Specifications

☐ Adult/child CPAP

   ☐ Continuous flow system   _____

   ☐ Demand flow system   _____

☐ Adult/child PEEP

   ☐ Continuous flow system   _____

   ☐ Demand flow system   _____

    ☐ Infant/neonatal CPAP

       ☐ Continuous flow system   _____

          ☐ Mask   _____

          ☐ Endotracheal tube   _____

          ☐ Nasal prongs   _____

       ☐ Demand flow system

          ☐ Mask   _____

          ☐ Endotracheal tube   _____

          ☐ Nasal prongs   _____

Other equipment specifications: _____

_____

_____

V. Outcome Criteria

The goals of instituting continuous distending pressure therapy, where possible, should be achieved without untoward patient response.

VI. Oral Review Questions

A. Adult CPAP/PEEP

1. What are the clinical indications, desirable and undesirable physiological effects, contraindications, and hazards of continuous distending pressure therapy in adults?

2. Describe the mechanism by which PEEP/CPAP is developed and maintained with the system being employed. Explain any/all alarm functions/indications.

3. Explain the concept of "optimum PEEP/CPAP." Provide all necessary equations or explain methods of assessment and interpretation of both subjective observations and objective data. Relate this concept to the patient under care (clinical setting only).

B. Neonatal/Pediatric CPAP

   1. Differentiate between the clinical indications, desirable and
      undesirable physiological effects, contraindications and
      hazards of CPAP applied to neonates as compared to adult
      applications.
   2. Describe the principle of operation, advantages,
      disadvantages, and limitations of the following techniques
      of generating CPAP;
         flow resistor systems (e.g., Gregory)
         threshold resistor systems

II. BEHAVIORAL RATING SCALES

INTRODUCTION

The demonstration of technical proficiency, as assessed by the proficiency evaluations in Section I, is necessary but insufficient evidence of competency attainment. Procedural expertise and knowledge alone cannot guarantee success as a respiratory care practitioner. The competent professional continually strives to integrate technical proficiency with consistent patterns of effective behavior. Ultimately, such behavior complements one's technical expertise and assures that the overall quality of services provided by the practitioner meets the expectations of consumers, providers, and the profession alike. The methods and procedures for assessing your ability to demonstrate the key components of professional behavior are included in this section of the manual.

SETTING

Whereas the proficiency evaluations described in Section I focus on discrete and easily isolated elements of competency, the assessment of professional behavior requires a more global approach. Professional behavior represents a complex synthesis of attributes that simply cannot be developed, demonstrated, or evaluated on a piecemeal basis. Valid and reliable determinations of the extent to which you exhibit behaviors consistent with professional expectations can only be accomplished by continuing observation of your real-life performance over time.

In regard to setting, the development and assessment of your professional behaviors will therefore take place whenever and wherever the opportunity exists to display such expectations, i.e., throughout your clinical learning experience. Such a holistic perspective ensures that sufficient opportunities will be available for you to develop and demonstrate the appropriate behaviors and that evaluation of these behaviors will result in reliable and valid judgments of your performance.

Methods and Procedures

Format. The format for evaluation of your professional behavior is necessarily different from that employed to assess your technical proficiency. The "checklist" format used for your proficiency evaluations is based upon determination of the presence or absence of satisfactory performance on particular steps in a given procedure. Similarly, summary judgments of your overall proficiency on a given skill take an either/or form, i.e., your performance is judged as either satisfactory or unsatisfactory. This all-or-nothing approach is clearly inappropriate for assessing your professional behavior.

The traits constituting professional behavior are observed in degrees. Quantification of such traits must therefore focus either on how much of a given characteristic is present or how well it is exhibited or performed. A graduated method of quantifying a behavioral trait is called a rating scale. When something as complex as professional behavior is being evaluated, many such scales, each evaluating a separate trait or attribute, are combined into a single comprehensive instrument. Your development and demonstration of professional behavior will be assessed using one or more forms of a comprehensive, multiattribute rating scale.

Professional attributes. The attributes chosen for inclusion in the rating scales that follow represent those identified by consensus among a sample of respiratory therapy educators, managers, and clinical practitioners as necessary for effective entry-level practice. The 20 discrete attributes constituting each scale provide both the specifications for and methods of assessing four major components of your professional behavior: (1) reasoning ability, (2) work performance, (3) interpersonal skills, and (4) personal characteristics.

The component of professional behavior labeled reasoning ability includes attribute ratings of your intellectual capacity, i.e., your knowledge, comprehension, theory integration, and learning adaptability. Judgments on the extent to which you demonstrate these attributes will commonly be drawn, in part, from concurrent ratings of your technical knowledge, as demonstrated during the oral review component of the proficiency evaluations. Other sources of information useful in making judgments regarding your reasoning ability include observations of your verbal interaction during clinical demonstrations, bedside rounds, case conferences, and other related situations in which the opportunity to demonstrate your learning arises.

The component of professional behavior labeled work performance consists of attribute ratings of the effectiveness with which you discharge your job role. Although your role as a student in the clinical setting is not totally equivalent to the expectations set for the employed practitioner, several attributes of your behavior, particularly in the latter stages of your clinical experience, are job-related. Included in this category are ratings of the quality and quantity of your performance, your judgment and organizational abilities, your observational acuity, and fulfillment of record-keeping and equipment maintenance responsibilities. Sources of information on which judgments of your work performance will be drawn will commonly include (but not be limited to) observations made during proficiency evaluations of your technical skills. Other pertinent sources of information on your work performance include more generalized observations of your behavior occurring under the supervised work experience phase(s) of your clinical education, i.e., during extended or full-time practicum rotations where you are delegated significant independent responsibilities.

The component of professional behavior labeled interpersonal skills includes attribute ratings of your ability to effectively interact with others, i.e., your general demeanor, communicative ability and attentiveness to patients' needs. Judgments on the extent to which you demonstrate these traits will be drawn from direct observations of your interactions with patients, peers, and professional colleagues. Such opportunities arise during therapeutic interventions at the bedside, during formal or informal interactions with the departmental, nursing, medical and ancillary staffs, and during group or individualized student learning activities.

The component of professional behavior labeled personal characteristics consists of attribute ratings of selected intrinsic traits that are volitional in nature, i.e., dependent upon your conscious choice and generally not constrained by external circumstances (as the other components can often be). Included in the category are ratings of your initiative, cooperativeness, dependability and self-direction, collaborativeness, integrity, punctuality, and personal appearance. Sources of information on which judgments of your personal characteristics will be drawn include essentially all of the observational opportunities previously identified for the other three components of professional behavior.

The rating procedure. Depending upon the methods employed by your program faculty, ratings of your professional behavior may be conducted for formative purposes, for summative purposes, or both.

Formative ratings of professional behavior are generally conducted at frequent intervals throughout your progression of clinical learning experiences. The purpose of formative evaluation is to help you clarify and develop those behaviors consistent with the expectations of your program and the local and professional communities it serves. Feedback provided by formative evaluation is generally not utilized in the determination of your clinical grade. In most situations, formative evaluation will be provided using the short form of the Behavioral Rating Scale.

Summative ratings of professional behavior are usually conducted at the end of a specific clinical unit, rotation, or course. The purpose of summative evaluation is to make a final or summary judgment of the extent to which your behaviors are consistent with the professional attributes previously described. The mechanism by which such summative evaluation(s) (where utilized) will be incorporated into the grading process will be described by your program faculty. In most situations, summative evaluations of your professional behavior will be determined using the long form of the Behavioral Rating Scale.

Regardless of the approach utilized, ratings of your professional behavior follow the same procedural steps, i.e., observation, documentation, rating, and review. The observation step occurs (as previously described) whenever and wherever the opportunity arises for you to exhibit the applicable attributes.

The documentation step requires supervisors, evaluators, and/or faculty to identify and describe in writing specific incidents of effective or ineffective behaviors, as related to the various scale attributes. Such incidents, when properly documented, are referred to as <u>critical incidents.</u>

At the end of the applicable time frame, the documented incidents are reviewed and judgments are drawn as to the extent or degree to which your behavior is consistent with each of the scale attributes. On the short form of the Behavioral Rating Scale, evaluators will indicate their judgments by specifying their degree of agreement with representative attribute statements. On the long form of the Behavioral Rating Scale, evaluators will choose, for each attribute, that statement corresponding most closely to your observed behavior. Because of the inherent variations common to the clinical education experience, both forms provide a mechanism to accommodate those circumstances in which a specific attribute is either not applicable or your evaluators had insufficient opportunity to observe the applicable behavior.

The review phase of the rating process provides you with an opportunity to go over both the ratings themselves and their supporting documentation. For formative purposes, the review step assures that you receive meaningful feedback regarding your professional behavior, i.e., that areas of strength and/or weakness be identified and that mechanisms be developed to capitalize upon your strengths and (where necessary) remediate your weaknesses. For summative purposes, the review phase provides you with the opportunity to review supporting documentation and assess (from your perspective) both its accuracy and the appropriateness of the resultant judgments.

Expectations regarding the degree to which your behavior should be consistent with the various scale attributes will be set by your program faculty. They may "average" scale scores as a whole, apply "average" scores to each of the four major scale components, or require a set level of behavior for each of the 20 discrete attributes. Regardless of the mechanism used, it is essential that you be clear as to exactly what your program's expectations are, and how they will be applied in the evaluation process.

Student Responsibilities

Your success in the development and demonstration of appropriate professional behaviors is dependent, in part, upon fulfilling three major responsibilities: (1) developing a clear knowledge of your program's behavioral expectations, (2) striving continually to demonstrate behaviors consistent with such expectations, and (3) ensuring that all relevant behaviors are accurately described and properly documented by those responsible for your evaluation.

Developing a knowledge of your program's behavioral expectations requires that you carefully review the attribute descriptions (or modifications thereof) included in the Behavioral Rating Scales. With its detailed description of each attribute, the long form of the scale is particularly useful for this purpose. Additional insight can be obtained by asking your program personnel to provide examples of particularly effective or ineffective behaviors, as related to specific scale attributes.

Given a clear understanding of such expectations, it is incumbent upon you to continually apply the appropriate behaviors whenever and wherever the opportunities arise. Although this may, in the early stages of your clinical experience, require deliberate forethought, such behaviors commonly become incorporated into a consistent pattern of performance, needing little conscious attention.

Developing such a pattern of performance is, of course, essential. Only those behaviors that are observed, accurately described, and properly documented, however, contribute to your evaluation. For this reason, it is crucial that you participate as an active partner in the evaluation of your professional behavior, drawing attention to relevant episodes or incidents , encouraging evaluators to document them, and carefully reviewing all resultant documentation and judgments. Certainly, differences in opinion and variations in interpretation regarding your behavior can and will occur—no rating process can be entirely objective. Without your input, however, neither the formative nor summative processes described can be expected to fully achieve their intended purpose—assisting you in developing a consistent pattern of professional behavior.

BEHAVIORAL RATING SCALE (SHORT FORM)

STUDENT	HOSPITAL/ROTATION
COURSE/UNIT	DATE(S)

INSTRUCTIONS: Please be frank and honest in reacting to the following statements regarding your opinion of the student's clinical performance. Circle the appropriate response. SA means you strongly agree; A means you agree; U means you are undecided; D means you disagree; and NA means not applicable or not observed.

THE STUDENT   RATING

1. Initiates unambiguous and goal-directed communication   SA   A   U   D   SD   NA

2. Establishes priorities and efficiently plans
   activities/assignments   SA   A   U   D   SD   NA

3. Displays adequate knowledge of essential concepts   SA   A   U   D   SD   NA

4. Exhibits courteous and pleasant demeanor   SA   A   U   D   SD   NA

5. Demonstrates thoroughness and attention to safety
   requirements   SA   A   U   D   SD   NA

6. Reports on patient's status/needs by observation and
   assessment   SA   A   U   D   SD   NA

7. Exhibits self-direction and responsibility for actions   SA   A   U   D   SD   NA

8. Displays cooperativeness and receptivity to suggestions
   and ideas   SA   A   U   D   SD   NA

9. Maintains concise and accurate records   SA   A   U   D   SD   NA

10. Presents a well-groomed and tidy personal appearance   SA   A   U   D   SD   NA

11. Grasps new experiences and readily adjusts to changing
    conditions   SA   A   U   D   SD   NA

12. Provides for adequate care and maintenance of equipment
    and supplies   SA   A   U   D   SD   NA

13. Displays forthrightness and integrity in dealings with
    patients and peers   SA   A   U   D   SD   NA

14. Accepts and applies supervisory guidance and
    constructive criticism   SA   A   U   D   SD   NA

15. Demonstrates the relationship(s) between theory and
    clinical practice   SA   A   U   D   SD   NA

16. Completes delegated tasks and assignments on schedule   SA   A   U   D   SD   NA

17. Seeks out new or additional activities on own
    initiative   SA   A   U   D   SD   NA

18. Demonstrates consideration and respect for patient's
    needs/rights   SA   A   U   D   SD   NA

19. Follows directions and exhibits sound judgment   SA   A   U   D   SD   NA

20. Displays punctuality and dependable adherence to time
    schedules   SA   A   U   D   SD   NA

OBSERVATIONS AND RECOMMENDATIONS

DATE	CRITICAL INCIDENT DESCRIPTIONS: Include (where applicable) the events leading up to the incident (antecedents), the behavior itself, and any observed consequences of the behavior. Be as specific and objective as possible.	APPLICABLE STATEMENT

COMMENTS AND IMPRESSIONS	RECOMMENDATIONS

EVALUATOR	FACULTY	STUDENT

BEHAVIORAL RATING SCALE (LONG FORM)

STUDENT	HOSPITAL/AFFILIATE
ROTATION	DATES

PARTICIPATING EVALUATORS

OVERALL RATING

REASONING ABILITY	INTERPERSONAL SKILLS
WORK PERFORMANCE	PERSONAL CHARACTERISTICS

COMMENTS AND IMPRESSIONS

RECOMMENDATIONS

STUDENT	EVALUATOR(S)	FACULTY

OBSERVATIONS

DATE	CRITICAL INCIDENT DESCRIPTIONS: Include (where applicable) the events leading up to the incident (antecedents), the behavior itself, and any observed consequences of the behavior. Be as specific and objective as possible.	APPLICABLE SCALE(S)

BEHAVIORAL RATING SCALE (LONG FORM)

	VERBAL COMMUNICATION
	CARRIES ON CONSISTENTLY GOAL-DIRECTED COMMUNICATION; IS ALWAYS DEFINITE, UNAMBIGUOUS, AND CLEAR IN MEANING AND INTENT.
	USUALLY INITIATES GOAL-DIRECTED COMMUNICATION THAT IS INFORMED, DELIBERATE, AND GENERALLY UNAMBIGUOUS.
	GENERALLY INITIATES ADEQUATE COMMUNICATION WITH INFREQUENT ERRORS OF INDEFINITENESS OR AMBIGUITY; SELDOM DISPLAYS MISLEADING WORD CHOICES OR ILLFORMIDNESS.
	OFTEN HAS DIFFICULTY IN COMMUNICATING MEANING OR INTENT; IS FREQUENTLY AMBIGUOUS OR INDEFINITE; OFTEN CHOOSES MISLEADING WORDS OR EXHIBITS ILLFORMIDNESS.
	IS CONSISTENTLY AMBIGUOUS AND INDEFINITE; MISLEADING WORDS OR LACK OF CLARITY IN INTENT AND MEANING PRECLUDE EFFECTIVE COMMUNICATION.
	AT PRESENT THERE IS INSUFFICIENT INFORMATION AVAILABLE TO PROVIDE A VALID RATING; OR, THIS SCALE IS NOT APPLICABLE (CIRCLE APPROPRIATE STATEMENT).

COMMENTS (CITE SPECIFIC INCIDENTS FROM WHICH THE ABOVE CONCLUSIONS WERE DRAWN)

	ORGANIZATION AND EFFICIENCY
	ALWAYS SETS GOALS AND PLANS AND ORGANIZES ACTIVITIES SO AS TO ACHIEVE OPTIMUM AND EFFICIENT PATIENT CARE.
	ORGANIZES AND PLANS ASSIGNMENTS WELL; FAILS TO ACHIEVE ESTABLISHED GOALS ONLY WHEN UNEXPECTED CIRCUMSTANCES INTERVENE.
	USUALLY ESTABLISHES PRIORITIES AND PLANS ACTIVITIES EFFICIENTLY; MOST GOALS ACHIEVED AS INTENDED.
	MAKES SOME ATTEMPT TO SET GOALS AND ORGANIZE ACTIVITIES BUT MANY PRIORITIES ARE NOT ACHIEVED.
	EXHIBITS NO PLANNING OR GOAL SETTING; IS UNAWARE OF PRIORITIES AND IS CONSTANTLY DISORGANIZED.
	AT PRESENT THERE IS INSUFFICIENT INFORMATION AVAILABLE TO PROVIDE A VALID RATING; OR, THIS SCALE IS NOT APPLICABLE (CIRCLE APPROPRIATE STATEMENT).

COMMENTS (CITE SPECIFIC INCIDENTS FROM WHICH THE ABOVE CONCLUSIONS WERE DRAWN)

BEHAVIORAL RATING SCALE (LONG FORM)

KNOWLEDGE AND COMPREHENSION

	DEMONSTRATES SUPERIOR COMPREHENSION AND KNOWLEDGE BEYOND THE REQUIREMENTS OF THE JOB.
	DEMONSTRATES ABOVE AVERAGE KNOWLEDGE AND COMPREHENSION BEYOND THAT ESSENTIAL.
	DISPLAYS ADEQUATE KNOWLEDGE OF ESSENTIAL CONCEPTS.
	HAS LIMITED UNDERSTANDING OF BASIC CONCEPTS; IS UNSURE OF ESSENTIALS.
	DISPLAYS INADEQUATE COMPREHENSION OF EVEN BASIC KNOWLEDGE.
	AT PRESENT THERE IS INSUFFICIENT INFORMATION AVAILABLE TO PROVIDE A VALID RATING; OR, THIS SCALE IS NOT APPLICABLE (CIRCLE APPROPRIATE STATEMENT).

COMMENTS (CITE SPECIFIC INCIDENTS FROM WHICH THE ABOVE CONCLUSIONS WERE DRAWN)

GENERAL DEMEANOR

	ALWAYS PLEASANT, COURTEOUS, FRIENDLY, AND TACTFUL; FOSTERS POSITIVE RESPONSE IN OTHERS.
	GENERALLY PLEASANT AND COURTEOUS; IS POISED, ACCEPTING, AND TACTFUL MOST OF THE TIME.
	USUALLY COURTEOUS AND PLEASANT; EXHIBITS TACTLESSNESS OR ABRUPTNESS ONLY IN EXTENUATING CIRCUMSTANCES.
	ABRUPT AND ANXIOUS AT TIMES, OFTEN DETACHED OR UNRESPONSIVE; MUST BE REMINDED OCCASIONALLY TO BE TACTFUL AND COURTEOUS.
	REGULARLY ABRUPT, RUDE, DOMINEERING, UNACCEPTING, OR CONDESCENDING; REQUIRES CONSTANT REMINDER TO DISPLAY TACT, COURTESY, OR UNDERSTANDING.
	AT PRESENT THERE IS INSUFFICIENT INFORMATION AVAILABLE TO PROVIDE A VALID RATING; OR, THIS SCALE IS NOT APPLICABLE (CIRCLE APPROPRIATE STATEMENT).

COMMENTS (CITE SPECIFIC INCIDENTS FROM WHICH THE ABOVE CONCLUSIONS WERE DRAWN)

BEHAVIORAL RATING SCALE (LONG FORM)

	THOROUGHNESS AND SAFETY
	CONSISTENTLY DEMONSTRATES THOROUGHNESS, ACCURACY, ATTENTION TO DETAIL; PERFORMANCE EXCEEDS SAFETY EXPECTATIONS AND IS ESSENTIALLY ERROR-FREE.
	USUALLY EXHIBITS THOROUGHNESS; WORK SELDOM NEEDS TO BE RECHECKED; DEMONSTRATES DUE CONSIDERATION FOR SAFETY AND ERRORS ARE FEW.
	DEMONSTRATES AN ACCEPTABLE LEVEL OF PERFORMANCE WITH OCCASIONAL (THOUGH NOT CRITICAL) ERRORS; SAFETY CONSIDERATIONS ARE RARELY OVERLOOKED.
	IS FREQUENTLY CARELESS OR NEGLIGENT, LACKING ATTENTION TO MANY DETAILS; ERRORS OCCUR FREQUENTLY AND SAFETY CONSIDERATIONS ARE OFTEN OVERLOOKED; REQUIRES CLOSE SUPERVISION.
	EXHIBITS OVERT CARELESSNESS AND CONSISTENTLY POOR QUALITY OF PERFORMANCE; MAKES CRITICAL ERRORS OF POTENTIAL DANGER TO PATIENT'S WELL-BEING; IS UNSAFE AND HAZARDOUS.
	AT PRESENT THERE IS INSUFFICIENT INFORMATION AVAILABLE TO PROVIDE A VALID RATING; OR, THIS SCALE IS NOT APPLICABLE (CIRCLE APPROPRIATE STATEMENT)

COMMENTS (CITE SPECIFIC INCIDENTS FROM WHICH THE ABOVE CONCLUSIONS WERE DRAWN)

	OBSERVATION, ASSESSMENT, REPORTING OF PATIENT'S STATUS/NEEDS
	CONSISTENTLY ASTUTE AND CONSCIENTIOUS IN THE OBSERVATION, ASSESSMENT, AND REPORTING OF PATIENT'S STATUS OR NEEDS TO APPROPRIATE PERSONNEL.
	USUALLY ALERT TO MOST CHANGES, NEVER OVERLOOKS OR FAILS TO REPORT PATIENT'S CONDITION OR NEEDS TO APPROPRIATE PERSONNEL.
	PROVIDES SATISFACTORY OBSERVATION AND ASSESSMENT OF PATIENT'S STATUS AND NEEDS; GENERALLY ASSURES THAT APPROPRIATE PERSONNEL ARE NOTIFIED.
	IS OFTEN CARELESS IN OBSERVING AND ASSESSING PATIENT'S CONDITION OR NEEDS; OFTEN FAILS TO COMMUNICATE CHANGES TO APPROPRIATE PERSONNEL.
	HABITUALLY DISPLAYS NEGLIGENCE IN PATIENT OBSERVATION AND ASSESSMENT; DOES NOT INFORM APPROPRIATE PERSONNEL OF PATIENT'S STATUS OR NEEDS.
	AT PRESENT THERE IS INSUFFICIENT INFORMATION AVAILABLE TO PROVIDE A VALID RATING; OR, THIS SCALE IS NOT APPLICABLE (CIRCLE APPROPRIATE STATEMENT).

COMMENTS (CITE SPECIFIC INCIDENTS FROM WHICH THE ABOVE CONCLUSIONS WERE DRAWN)

BEHAVIORAL RATING SCALE (LONG FORM)

	DEPENDABILITY AND SELF-DIRECTION
	ASSUMES FULL RESPONSIBILITY FOR ACTIONS AND EXHIBITS SELF-DIRECTION IN ALL ACTIVITIES; CAN INDEPENDENTLY INITIATE POSITIVE ACTION AND RARELY REQUIRES DIRECT SUPERVISION.
	IS GENERALLY ABLE TO ASSUME RESPONSIBILITY FOR ACTIONS; USUALLY INITIATES INDEPENDENT ACTION AND SELF-DIRECTION; REQUIRES MINIMAL SUPERVISION.
	IS DEPENDABLE AND SELF-DIRECTED IN ASSUMING MOST RESPONSIBILITIES; IS AWARE OF LIMITATIONS AND SEEKS SUPERVISION AND ASSISTANCE WHEN NECESSARY.
	RELUCTANT TO ASSUME SELF-DIRECTION OR INDEPENDENTLY INITIATE ACTIONS; REQUIRES CLOSE OBSERVATION AND SUPERVISION IN MOST ACTIVITIES.
	CANNOT ASSUME RESPONSIBILITY FOR ACTIONS; LACKS DIRECTION AND REQUIRES CONSTANT OBSERVATION AND DIRECT SUPERVISION.
	AT PRESENT THERE IS INSUFFICIENT INFORMATION AVAILABLE TO PROVIDE A VALID RATING; OR, THIS SCALE IS NOT APPLICABLE (CIRCLE APPROPRIATE STATEMENT).

COMMENTS (CITE SPECIFIC INCIDENTS FROM WHICH THE ABOVE CONCLUSIONS WERE DRAWN)

	COOPERATIVENESS AND RECEPTIVENESS
	EXCEPTIONALLY COOPERATIVE AND RECEPTIVE TO SUGGESTIONS AND NEW IDEAS.
	HIGHLY RESPONSIVE AND COOPERATIVE; GENERALLY RECEPTIVE TO SUGGESTIONS AND NEW IDEAS.
	USUALLY COOPERATES, DOES NOT RESIST NEW IDEAS. SELDOM FAILS TO TAKE SUGGESTIONS.
	UNRESPONSIVE AT TIMES, OFTEN FAILING TO COOPERATE; RESISTS NEW IDEAS AND SELDOM CARRIES OUT SUGGESTIONS.
	IS HABITUALLY UNCOOPERATIVE AND UNRECEPTIVE; RESENTS OR REJECTS SUGGESTIONS AND NEW IDEAS.
	AT PRESENT THERE IS INSUFFICIENT INFORMATION AVAILABLE TO PROVIDE A VALID RATING; OR, THIS SCALE IS NOT APPLICABLE (CIRCLE APPROPRIATE STATEMENT).

COMMENTS (CITE SPECIFIC INCIDENTS FROM WHICH THE ABOVE CONCLUSIONS WERE DRAWN)

BEHAVIORAL RATING SCALE (LONG FORM)

	RECORD KEEPING
	ALWAYS MAINTAINS EXCEPTIONALLY COMPLETE, ACCURATE, AND CONCISE RECORDS IN FULL ACCORD WITH HOSPITAL AND DEPARTMENTAL POLICY AND PROCEDURES.
	ENSURES THAT RECORDS KEPT ARE COMPLETE AND CONCISE; RECOGNIZES AND CORRECTS ANY ERRORS OR OMISSIONS.
	USUALLY MAINTAINS RECORDS THAT ARE SATISFACTORY; OCCASIONALLY MAKES MINOR ERRORS OR FAILS TO PROVIDE COMPLETE DESCRIPTION OF ACTIONS/ASSESSMENTS.
	IS FREQUENTLY CARELESS IN COMPLETING PROPER RECORDS; COMMITS MANY ERRORS OR IS OFTEN INACCURATE AND INCOMPLETE.
	HABITUALLY FAILS TO PROVIDE DOCUMENTATION OF ACTIVITIES.
	AT PRESENT THERE IS INSUFFICIENT INFORMATION AVAILABLE TO PROVIDE A VALID RATING; OR, THIS SCALE IS NOT APPLICABLE (CIRCLE APPROPRIATE STATEMENT).

COMMENTS (CITE SPECIFIC INCIDENTS FROM WHICH THE ABOVE CONCLUSIONS WERE DRAWN)

	PERSONAL APPEARANCE
	ALWAYS PRESENTS A CLEAN AND WELL-GROOMED APPEARANCE THAT EXCEEDS THE BASIC DRESS CODE REQUIREMENTS.
	CONSISTENTLY NEAT AND WELL-GROOMED IN ACCORD WITH BASIC DRESS REQUIREMENTS.
	USUALLY PRESENTS CLEAN AND SATISFACTORY APPEARANCE, RARELY UNTIDY OR INAPPROPRIATE.
	OFTEN FORGETFUL OF STANDARDS OF APPEARANCE OR GROOMING, AT TIMES UNTIDY OR INAPPROPRIATELY DRESSED.
	HABITUALLY NEGLIGENT OF APPEARANCE; CONSISTENTLY UNTIDY, UNKEMPT, OR UNCLEAN.
	AT PRESENT THERE IS INSUFFICIENT INFORMATION AVAILABLE TO PROVIDE A VALID RATING; OR, THIS SCALE IS NOT APPLICABLE (CIRCLE APPROPRIATE STATEMENT).

COMMENTS (CITE SPECIFIC INCIDENTS FROM WHICH THE ABOVE CONCLUSIONS WERE DRAWN)

BEHAVIORAL RATING SCALE (LONG FORM)

LEARNING ADAPTABILITY

	LEARNS AND APPLIES NEW EXPERIENCES EXCEPTIONALLY QUICKLY; ADJUSTS RAPIDLY TO NEW CONDITIONS OR ALTERED SITUATIONS.
	IS RATHER QUICK TO LEARN FROM NEW EXPERIENCES; READILY ACCOMMODATES CHANGED CONDITIONS OR SITUATIONS.
	GRASPS NEW EXPERIENCES AND ADJUSTS TO CHANGES WHEN GIVEN A SATISFACTORY TIME INTERVAL.
	IS RATHER SLOW IN LEARNING NEW TASKS AND HAS SOME DIFFICULTY ACCOMMODATING TO CHANGING CONDITIONS.
	SEEMS UNABLE TO LEARN FROM OR APPLY NEW EXPERIENCES AND CANNOT ADJUST TO CHANGES.
	AT PRESENT THERE IS INSUFFICIENT INFORMATION AVAILABLE TO PROVIDE A VALID RATING; OR, THIS SCALE IS NOT APPLICABLE (CIRCLE APPROPRIATE STATEMENT).

COMMENTS (CITE SPECIFIC INCIDENTS FROM WHICH THE ABOVE CONCLUSIONS WERE DRAWN)

CARE AND USE OF EQUIPMENT AND/OR SUPPLIES

	DEMONSTRATES EXEMPLARY COMPETENCE AND RESOURCEFULNESS IN THE UTILIZATION AND CARE OF EQUIPMENT AND SUPPLIES.
	EFFICIENTLY EMPLOYS AVAILABLE EQUIPMENT AND SUPPLIES, GIVING DUE CARE TO THEIR USE AND MAINTENANCE.
	EXHIBITS SATISFACTORY CARE AND USE OF EQUIPMENT IN MOST SITUATIONS; IS NEVER NEGLIGENT, WASTEFUL, OR ABUSIVE.
	IS OFTEN INEFFICIENT IN THE USE OR MAINTENANCE OF EQUIPMENT AND OCCASIONALLY PROVIDES LESS THAN ADEQUATE CARE.
	IS ABUSIVE, NEGLIGENT, AND CARELESS IN THE USE AND CARE OF EQUIPMENT OR SUPPLIES.
	AT PRESENT THERE IS INSUFFICIENT INFORMATION AVAILABLE TO PROVIDE A VALID RATING; OR, THIS SCALE IS NOT APPLICABLE (CIRCLE APPROPRIATE STATEMENT).

COMMENTS (CITE SPECIFIC INCIDENTS FROM WHICH THE ABOVE CONCLUSIONS WERE DRAWN)

BEHAVIORAL RATING SCALE (LONG FORM)

INTEGRITY
CONSISTENTLY EXHIBITS CONCERN FOR THE DIGNITY AND WELFARE OF PATIENTS AND ENSURES CONFIDENCE OF PRIVILEGED INFORMATION; ALWAYS ACKNOWLEDGES LIMITATIONS OF PRACTICE AND RESPONSIBILITY/AUTHORITY GRANTED BY THE PHYSICIAN; MAINTAINS FORTHRIGHT AND HONEST BEHAVIOR AT ALL TIMES.
GENERALLY DISPLAYS CONCERN FOR THE DIGNITY AND WELFARE OF PATIENTS AND ENSURES CONFIDENCE OF PRIVILEGED INFORMATION; GENERALLY RECOGNIZES LIMITATIONS OF PRACTICE AND RESPONSIBILITY/AUTHORITY GRANTED BY THE PHYSICIAN; CONSISTENTLY DISPLAYS FORTHRIGHT BEHAVIOR.
SELDOM FAILS TO RECOGNIZE THE IMPORTANCE OF THE PATIENT'S DIGNITY AND WELFARE AND RESPONSIBILITY OF PRIVILEGED COMMUNICATION; USUALLY RECOGNIZES LIMITATION OF PRACTICE AND RESPONSIBILITY/AUTHORITY GRANTED BY THE PHYSICIAN; USUALLY DISPLAYS FORTHRIGHT AND HONEST BEHAVIOR.
OFTEN DISREGARDS PATIENT'S DIGNITY OR WELFARE AND RIGHT TO PRIVILEGED COMMUNI-CATION; IS SOMETIMES NEGLIGENT IN ACKNOWLEDGING LIMITATIONS OF PRACTICE AND RESPONSIBILITY/AUTHORITY GRANTED BY THE PHYSICIAN; FAILS AT TIMES TO BE FORTHRIGHT AND HONEST.
IS NEGLIGENT OR ABUSIVE OF PATIENT'S DIGNITY AND CONSISTENTLY FAILS TO MAINTAIN CONFIDENTIALITY OF PRIVILEGED COMMUNICATIONS; FAILS TO RECOGNIZE LIMITATIONS TO PRACTICE AND IS ABUSIVE OF RESPONSIBILITY/AUTHORITY GRANTED BY PHYSICIAN; IS OFTEN DISHONEST.
AT PRESENT THERE IS INSUFFICIENT INFORMATION AVAILABLE TO PROVIDE A VALID RATING; OR, THIS SCALE IS NOT APPLICABLE (CIRCLE APPROPRIATE STATEMENT).
COMMENTS (CITE SPECIFIC INCIDENTS FROM WHICH THE ABOVE CONCLUSIONS WERE DRAWN)

COLLABORATIVENESS
CONSISTENTLY COLLABORATES WITH SUPERVISORS AND INSTRUCTORS TO MAXIMIZE LEARNING AND IMPLEMENT OPTIMUM PATIENT CARE.
REACTS POSITIVELY TOWARDS GUIDANCE AND APPLIES SUPERVISORS' RECOMMENDATION TO IMPROVE KNOWLEDGE, SKILLS, OR ATTITUDES.
WILLINGLY ACCEPTS SUPERVISION AND GUIDANCE; GENERALLY APPLIES RECOMMENDATIONS AND IS RECEPTIVE TO CONSTRUCTIVE CRITICISM.
SOMETIMES REACTS NEGATIVELY TOWARDS SUPERVISION; OFTEN REJECTS GUIDANCE OR FAILS TO APPLY RECOMMENDATIONS; HAS DIFFICULTY ACCEPTING CONSTRUCTIVE CRITICISM.
RESENTS SUPERVISION AND REJECTS GUIDANCE; IS DEFENSIVE OR ABUSIVE WHEN APPROACHED WITH RECOMMENDATIONS; FAILS TO ALTER BEHAVIOR WHEN APPROPRIATENESS CRITICIZED.
AT PRESENT THERE IS INSUFFICIENT INFORMATION AVAILABLE TO PROVIDE A VALID RATING; OR, THIS SCALE IS NOT APPLICABLE (CIRCLE APPROPRIATE STATEMENT).
COMMENTS (CITE SPECIFIC INCIDENTS FROM WHICH THE ABOVE CONCLUSIONS WERE DRAWN)

BEHAVIORAL RATING SCALE (LONG FORM)

	THEORY INTEGRATION
	READILY TRANSFERS THEORETICAL KNOWLEDGE TO ALL CLINICAL SITUATIONS.
	APPLIES AND RELATES THEORY TO MOST CLINICAL ACTIVITIES.
	CAN USUALLY DEMONSTRATE HOW ESSENTIAL ASPECTS OF THEORY RELATE TO SPECIFIC CLINICAL SITUATIONS.
	EXHIBITS A SUPERFICIAL UNDERSTANDING OF THE APPLICATION OF THEORY IN MOST CLINICAL ACTIVITIES.
	IS UNAWARE OF AND CANNOT INTEGRATE THEORETICAL CONCEPTS WITH THEIR PRACTICAL APPLICATION.
	AT PRESENT THERE IS INSUFFICIENT INFORMATION AVAILABLE TO PROVIDE A VALID RATING; OR, THIS SCALE IS NOT APPLICABLE (CIRCLE APPROPRIATE STATEMENT).

COMMENTS (CITE SPECIFIC INCIDENTS FROM WHICH THE ABOVE CONCLUSIONS WERE DRAWN)

	QUANTITY OF PERFORMANCE
	WORKS CONSISTENTLY AND WITH EXCELLENT OUTPUT, UTILIZES TIME EFFICIENTLY.
	WORKS CONSISTENTLY WITH ABOVE AVERAGE OUTPUT; ALWAYS COMPLETES ASSIGNED FUNCTIONS IN APPROPRIATE TIME INTERVAL.
	MAINTAINS SATISFACTORY OUTPUT; IS USUALLY ABLE TO COMPLETE DELEGATED TASKS IN APPROPRIATE TIME INTERVAL.
	FREQUENTLY IS UNABLE TO COMPLETE ASSIGNED FUNCTIONS WITHIN A SATISFACTORY TIME LIMIT.
	DEMONSTRATES UNREALISTICALLY LOW OUTPUT IN RELATION TO EXPECTATIONS; IS SLOW AND HABITUALLY INEFFICIENT.
	AT PRESENT THERE IS INSUFFICIENT INFORMATION AVAILABLE TO PROVIDE A VALID RATING; OR, THIS SCALE IS NOT APPLICABLE (CIRCLE APPROPRIATE STATEMENT).

COMMENTS (CITE SPECIFIC INCIDENTS FROM WHICH THE ABOVE CONCLUSIONS WERE DRAWN)

BEHAVIORAL RATING SCALE (LONG FORM)

	INITIATIVE
	EXHIBITS ENTHUSIASM AND INITIATIVE IN PERFORMING ASSIGNED TASKS; CONTINUALLY SEEKS OUT NEW LEARNING EXPERIENCES BEYOND THOSE SCHEDULED OR PLANNED.
	READILY ACCEPTS ASSIGNED ACTIVITIES AND CONSTRUCTIVELY EXPLOITS THEIR LEARNING POTENTIAL; GENERALLY SEEKS OUT NEW OR ADDITIONAL LEARNING EXPERIENCES.
	KEEPS PACE WITH REGULAR WORK ASSIGNMENTS AND OCCASIONALLY SEEKS OUT NEW ACTIVITIES.
	REQUIRES OCCASIONAL PRODDING TO KEEP UP WITH DELEGATED TASKS, RARELY USES TIME CONSTRUCTIVELY.
	MUST BE CONTINUOUSLY PRODDED TO MEET RESPONSIBILITIES; COMPLETES ASSIGNED ACTIVITIES ONLY BECAUSE THEY ARE REQUIRED; DOES NOT SEEK OUT NEW LEARNING EXPERIENCES.
	AT PRESENT THERE IS INSUFFICIENT INFORMATION AVAILABLE TO PROVIDE A VALID RATING; OR, THIS SCALE IS NOT APPLICABLE (CIRCLE APPROPRIATE STATEMENT).

COMMENTS (CITE SPECIFIC INCIDENTS FROM WHICH THE ABOVE CONCLUSIONS WERE DRAWN)

	PATIENT RAPPORT AND CONSIDERATION
	COMMUNICATES READILY WITH PATIENTS; ALWAYS ATTENTIVE TO THEIR EMOTIONS, NEEDS, RIGHTS, AND COMFORT; IS CONSISTENTLY CONSIDERATE, PATIENT, AND ACCOMMODATING.
	MAINTAINS GOOD RAPPORT WITH PATIENTS; RECOGNIZES THEIR RIGHTS AND ATTEMPTS TO ACCOMMODATE THEIR NEEDS; IS RESPECTFUL AND COURTEOUS.
	GENERALLY SENSITIVE TO PATIENTS' NEEDS AND RIGHTS IN PLANNING CARE; COMMUNICATES ADEQUATELY TO GAIN PATIENTS' CONFIDENCE AND IS USUALLY CONSIDERATE AND RESPECTFUL.
	OFTEN IGNORES OR IS INATTENTIVE TO PATIENTS' RIGHTS AND COMFORT; HAS DIFFICULTY COMMUNICATING SINCERITY OR CONSIDERATION; GENERALLY FAILS TO ACHIEVE RAPPORT WITH PATIENTS.
	IS INCOGNIZANT OF PATIENTS' NEEDS, RIGHTS, OR NECESSARY COMFORTS; FAILS TO ADEQUATELY COMMUNICATE WITH PATIENT; IS INSINCERE OR DETACHED.
	AT PRESENT THERE IS INSUFFICIENT INFORMATION AVAILABLE TO PROVIDE A VALID RATING; OR, THIS SCALE IS NOT APPLICABLE (CIRCLE APPROPRIATE STATEMENT).

COMMENTS (CITE SPECIFIC INCIDENTS FROM WHICH THE ABOVE CONCLUSIONS WERE DRAWN)

BEHAVIORAL RATING SCALE (LONG FORM)

	COMPREHENSION AND JUDGMENT
	GRASPS DIRECTIONS QUICKLY AND ACCURATELY; DISPLAYS OUTSTANDING USE OF JUDGMENT.
	READILY USES INSTRUCTIONS AND MAKES DECISIONS BASED UPON SOUND JUDGMENT.
	RARELY REQUIRES REPETITION OF EXPLANATIONS OR REFERRAL TO INSTRUCTIONS; DEMONSTRATES GOOD JUDGMENT IN MOST SITUATIONS.
	REQUIRES NEEDLESS RE-EXPLANATIONS; HAS DIFFICULTY IN MAKING RATIONAL JUDGMENTS.
	IS UNABLE TO FOLLOW EVEN SIMPLE DIRECTIONS; CANNOT BE DEPENDED UPON TO MAKE SOUND JUDGMENTS.
	AT PRESENT THERE IS INSUFFICIENT INFORMATION AVAILABLE TO PROVIDE A VALID RATING; OR, THIS SCALE IS NOT APPLICABLE (CIRCLE APPROPRIATE STATEMENT).

COMMENTS (CITE SPECIFIC INCIDENTS FROM WHICH THE ABOVE CONCLUSIONS WERE DRAWN)

	ATTENDANCE AND PUNCTUALITY
	IS NEVER ABSENT AND ALWAYS ARRIVES AS SCHEDULED (OR EARLY) FOR ALL ROTATIONS AND ACTIVITIES.
	IS ABSENT OR LATE ONLY UNDER EXTENUATING CIRCUMSTANCES AND WITH PROPER NOTIFICATION.
	IS RARELY ABSENT OR LATE FOR SCHEDULED ACTIVITIES; PROPERLY NOTIFIES APPROPRIATE PERSONNEL IN ADVANCE OF DIFFICULTIES IN ATTENDANCE; SEEKS TO MAKE UP LOST TIME.
	IS FREQUENTLY ABSENT OR TARDY AND OFTEN FAILS TO GIVE NOTIFICATION TO APPROPRIATE PERSONNEL; AVOIDS EFFORTS TO RESCHEDULE TIME.
	SHOWS DISDAIN FOR ATTENDANCE AND PUNCTUALITY REQUIREMENTS; HABITUALLY NEGLECTS TO GIVE NOTIFICATION; REJECTS EFFORTS TO RESCHEDULE LOST TIME.
	AT PRESENT THERE IS INSUFFICIENT INFORMATION AVAILABLE TO PROVIDE A VALID RATING; OR, THIS SCALE IS NOT APPLICABLE (CIRCLE APPROPRIATE STATEMENT).

COMMENTS (CITE SPECIFIC INCIDENTS FROM WHICH THE ABOVE CONCLUSIONS WERE DRAWN)

III. SUMMARY RECORDS

INTRODUCTION

The summary records included in this section provide the means to record and document your learning activities and assist both you and your faculty in monitoring your progress toward the achievement of clinical competency.

Methods and Procedures

Exactly which summary records will be employed by your faculty and how they will be utilized to record and document your progress will vary from program to program. The methods and procedures described in this section represent guidelines only. Specific instructions on the utilization of these summary records will be provided by your program faculty.

The Cumulative Proficiency Record. This record will normally be employed to document your achievement of proficiency in each of the 40 technical skills included in Section I of this manual. The Cumulative Proficiency Record lists these skills or procedures in the same order as they appear in Section I. For each procedure, space is provided to describe the setting, conditions, and equipment specifications under which your proficiency in performing that skill is to be evaluated. Normally, the conditions and equipment specifications will be directly transcribed onto this record from those provided by your instructors as they introduce or demonstrate each discrete skill. Alternatively, your faculty may provide a complete and detailed listing of these specifications during the early phases of your clinical education. In either case, provision has been made to specify, for each procedure, multiple variations in both the conditions under which your evaluation will occur and the equipment necessary for demonstrating proficiency.

The "Setting" columns of the Cumulative Proficiency Record also correspond to those designated in the Procedural Specifications component of each proficiency evaluation. Entries made in these columns will normally represent confirmation of the occurrence of a proficiency evaluation in the applicable setting, and, therefore, will usually be made only by your program faculty, clinical supervisors or evaluators, or their designees. Different programs will employ different mechanisms for coding entries in the setting columns; it is your responsibility to understand both how such entries will be made and their specific meaning.

In most programs, your faculty will maintain an official Cumulative Proficiency Record for each student on a duplicate form. Under these circumstances, the form provided in the manual serves as the personal (unofficial) record of your proficiency attainment. Where duplicate records are maintained, it is essential that entries be consistent with one another and accurately recorded in a timely fashion.

The Proficiency Assignment Form. This form will normally be employed by your faculty to specify the course, unit of instruction, clinical site, rotation, or time frame during which you are expected to complete specific proficiency evaluations. These assignments will usually be provided by your faculty at the beginning of each applicable unit of instruction or segment of clinical education. The careful delineation of proficiency evaluation assignments according to appropriate setting or time frame will provide you with clear expectations as to when and where such evaluations will occur and thus give you an opportunity to fulfill your preparatory responsibilities. Like the Cumulative Proficiency Record, the exact use of the Proficiency Assignment Form will be determined by your program faculty.

The Summary Evaluation and Recommendation Form. This form will normally be employed in those programs where faculty desire to combine assessment of technical skills and behavior in a comprehensive evaluation with, where necessary, appropriate recommendations. Under these circumstances, the Summary Evaluation and Recommendation Form would be utilized at the end of a specific clinical rotation, during which time you would have undergone both the assigned proficiency evaluations and the behavioral ratings applicable to that setting. Recommendations derived from your overall performance are thus based on your status in regard to both dimensions of clinical competency.

In terms of the technical skills assigned for the applicable rotation, you will have either (a) completed all proficiency evaluations with a satisfactory performance assessment, or (b) failed to complete all assigned proficiency evaluations (due to either performance errors or constraints beyond your control). In terms of the behavioral expectations set for the applicable rotation, your performance will have been judged either (a) satisfactory in all dimensions (as delineated by your faculty), or (b) unsatisfactory on some dimensions.

Combining these two overall assessments of competency into a single evaluation results in four possible status recommendations. Completion of all assigned proficiency evaluations and demonstration of satisfactory behavior on all applicable dimensions of professional behavior (Status 1) will normally indicate both successful achievement of the rotation's objectives and your readiness to proceed to subsequent assignments.

When you have demonstrated proficiency on all assigned technical skills, but one or more dimensions of your professional behavior are judged as unsatisfactory (Status 2), your faculty will make recommendations specific to those areas of behavior in question and will usually request that you meet with them to review their suggestions and jointly develop a plan to meet their expectations. Where the behavioral problems identified are minor or easily rectifiable, a subsequent satisfactory evaluation may be all that is required. Behavioral concerns of major consequence, however, particularly those affecting the safety or welfare of your patients, may jeopardize your clinical status and require immediate action and intensive remediation.

When your overall professional behavior is judged satisfactory, but, for whatever reason, you have failed to complete all assigned proficiency evaluations (Status 3), your faculty will normally require that you schedule additional clinical time to complete those evaluations on which your performance was deemed unsatisfactory or those for which circumstantial constraints prevented your fulfillment of the proficiency assignments. Incomplete proficiency evaluations may also be completed on subsequent rotations, thereby eliminating the necessity for additional clinical time. Some programs may also purposefully schedule "make-up" time as part of the clinical education experience. Regardless of the mechanism employed, programs using this "mastery" approach will expect that all students demonstrate proficiency on all assigned technical skills and procedures. Under these circumstances, your preparation for and practice of the applicable proficiencies prior to formal evaluation (see Section I) will minimize the need for remedial work and thus greatly expedite your progress toward competency attainment.

Where questions arise regarding both dimensions of professional competency, i.e., failure to complete the assigned proficiency evaluations, and unsatisfactory professional behavior (Status 4), your faculty will normally insist that you meet with them to review their recommendations and develop a plan whereby their concerns can be addressed and their expectations met. Such recommendations will usually be a combination of those applicable when either your proficiency evaluations are incomplete or your professional behavior judged unsatisfactory. As in these circumstances, the responsibility for meeting the faculty's expectations must ultimately be assumed by you.

The Clinical Log Form. This form represents a suggested format for recording and documenting your clinical learning experiences. Your program faculty may choose to use the form as provided, specify modifications in its format or usage, or provide alternative mechanisms to maintain a verifiable record of your clinical activity. The purpose of such documentation is twofold: to provide an individualized record of clinical learning experiences, and, to assist faculty in evaluating such experiences for equivalence. Scrutiny of your individual log entries provides a unique "picture" of your clinical experiences and their relevance to the applicable course, unit, or rotation objectives specified by your faculty. Reviewed together, these logs assist faculty in identifying the commonalities and differences in clinical experiences that occur among students, and can provide the basis for the sharing of important information or perspectives not otherwise available to the individual. It is for these reasons that the Clinical Log Form emphasizes activities other than those requiring formal evaluation, i.e., observational learning and physician contact. Moreover, the suggested format asks you to single out your most important daily learning experience(s) and elaborate upon their importance or significance to you and your peers. This particular activity, where required, can provide the basis for seminar-type discussions commonly employed in the latter phases of your formal clinical education.

The Laboratory Activity and Attendance Record. Where employed, this form provides a mechanism to briefly summarize your relevant laboratory activities and document your participation in this important setting. The form is particularly useful in those programs in which some or all of your laboratory experience is independently scheduled. Normally, the time entries will be verified by your laboratory supervisor(s) or, alternatively, by time-clock. In any case, you are responsible for utilizing the form (or modifications thereof) according to the specifications provided by your faculty.

Student Responsibilities

As emphasized throughout this manual, complete and accurate documentation is an essential prerequisite toward demonstrating the achievement of clinical competency. Just as you are expected to develop the skills and behavior necessary to competently deliver respiratory care to your patients, you are equally obliged to ensure that their development and achievement are thoroughly documented and accurately recorded.

The summary records provided in this Section of the manual have been designed to assist both you and your faculty in this complex and formidable task. Although their exact use will vary from program to program, the effectiveness of such records as tools for decision-making will ultimately depend upon the meticulousness and care you apply in their maintenance.

CUMULATIVE PROFICIENCY EVALUATION RECORD

PROCEDURE	CONDITIONS	EQUIPMENT	SETTING		
			LABORATORY	CLINIC	OTHER
VITAL SIGNS					
ARTERIAL BLOOD PRESSURE					
PATIENT POSITIONING					
PATIENT ASSESSMENT					

CUMULATIVE PROFICIENCY EVALUATION RECORD

PROCEDURE	CONDITIONS	EQUIPMENT	SETTING		
			LABORATORY	CLINIC	OTHER
MEDICAL RECORDS					
HAND-WASHING					
CHEMICAL DISINFECTION AND STERILIZATION					
GAS STERILIZATION					

CUMULATIVE PROFICIENCY EVALUATION RECORD

PROCEDURE	CONDITIONS	EQUIPMENT	SETTING		
			LABORATORY	CLINIC	OTHER
PASTEURIZATION					
BACTERIOLOGICAL SURVEILLANCE					
ISOLATION					
CYLINDER SAFETY AND TRANSPORT					

CUMULATIVE PROFICIENCY EVALUATION RECORD

PROCEDURE	CONDITIONS	EQUIPMENT	LABORATORY				CLINIC				OTHER			
OXYGEN THERAPY														
OXYHOOD														
MEASUREMENT OF OXYGEN CONCENTRATIONS														
AEROSOL/ HUMIDITY THERAPY														

CUMULATIVE PROFICIENCY EVALUATION RECORD

PROCEDURE	CONDITIONS	EQUIPMENT	SETTING		
			LABORATORY	CLINIC	OTHER
AEROSOL ENCLOSURES					
AEROSOL DRUG ADMINISTRATION					
INCENTIVE SPIROMETRY					
INTERMITTENT POSITIVE PRESSURE BREATHING					

CUMULATIVE PROFICIENCY EVALUATION RECORD

PROCEDURE	CONDITIONS	EQUIPMENT	SETTING		
			LABORATORY	CLINIC	OTHER
BREATHING EXERCISES					
COUGHING					
POSTURAL DRAINAGE AND PERCUSSION					
CARDIOPULMONARY RESUSCITATION (ADULT)					

CUMULATIVE PROFICIENCY EVALUATION RECORD

PROCEDURE	CONDITIONS	EQUIPMENT	SETTING		
			LABORATORY	CLINIC	OTHER
CARDIOPULMONARY RESUSCITATION (INFANT/CHILD)					
EMERGENCY ENDOTRACHEAL INTUBATION					
TRACHEOBRONCHIAL ASPIRATION					
CUFF MANAGEMENT					

CUMULATIVE PROFICIENCY EVALUATION RECORD

PROCEDURE	CONDITIONS	EQUIPMENT	SETTING			
			LABORATORY	CLINIC	OTHER	
TRACHEOSTOMY CARE						
ENDOTRACHEAL EXTUBATION						
BEDSIDE VENTILATORY ASSESSMENT						
FORCED EXPIRATORY VOLUME						

CUMULATIVE PROFICIENCY EVALUATION RECORD

PROCEDURE	CONDITIONS	EQUIPMENT	SETTING		
			LABORATORY	CLINIC	OTHER
FUNCTIONAL RESIDUAL CAPACITY					
DIFFUSING CAPACITY					
ARTERIAL BLOOD GAS SAMPLING					
ARTERIAL BLOOD GAS ANALYSIS					

323

CUMULATIVE PROFICIENCY EVALUATION RECORD

PROCEDURE	CONDITIONS	EQUIPMENT	SETTING									
			LABORATORY			CLINIC			OTHER			
VENTILATOR PREPARATION AND APPLICATION												
ROUTINE VENTILATOR CHECK												
IMV, WEANING, AND VENTILATOR DISCONTINUANCE												
CONTINUOUS DISTENDING PRESSURE THERAPY												

PROFICIENCY ASSIGNMENT FORM

COURSE OR UNIT OF INSTRUCTION	CLINICAL SITE OR ROTATION	APPLICABLE DATES OR TIMELINES	REQUIRED PROFICIENCY EVALUATIONS	SPECIAL INSTRUCTIONS OR COMMENTS

SUMMARY EVALUATION AND RECOMMENDATIONS

PROFICIENCY EVALUATIONS	BEHAVIORAL RATINGS
☐ INCOMPLETE ☐ COMPLETED (list below):	☐ UNSATISFACTORY ☐ SATISFACTORY (list below):

RECOMMENDATIONS

		PROFICIENCY EVALUATIONS	BEHAVIORAL RATINGS	RECOMMENDATIONS
S	1	Complete	Satisfactory	Rotation complete, progress to next assignment
T	2	Complete	Unsatisfactory	Review recommendations (below) and meet with faculty
A				
T	3	Incomplete	Satisfactory	Schedule additional clinical time for mastery or remediation of clinical skills
U				
S	4	Incomplete	Unsatisfactory	Review recommendations (below) and meet with faculty

SPECIFIC RECOMMENDATIONS:

STUDENT_____ FACULTY_____ EVALUATOR(S)_____

CLINICAL LOG FORM

HOSPITAL	DATE	SUPERVISOR (SIGNATURE)

PROCEDURES PERFORMED   COMMENTS:

OBSERVATIONS: COMMENTS:

PHYSICIAN CONTACT: ☐ FORMAL CLASS   ☐ BEDSIDE ROUNDS   ☐ OTHER (SPECIFY):
DESCRIBE NATURE AND ESTIMATE TIME:

DESCRIBE BRIEFLY THE MOST SIGNIFICANT LEARNING EXPERIENCE OCCURRING DURING THE DAY; USE ADDITIONAL DOCUMENTATION (GRAPHS, DRAWINGS, ETC.) IF NECESSARY SO THAT YOUR EXPERIENCE CAN BE SHARED WITH THE CLASS.

LABORATORY ACTIVITY AND ATTENDANCE RECORD

LABORATORY ACTIVITY (DEMONSTRATIONS, EXPERIMENTS, PRACTICE)	SUP. SIG	TIME RECORD (INC. DATE)
		IN
		OUT
		IN
		OUT
		IN
		OUT
		IN
		OUT
		IN
		OUT
		IN
		OUT
		IN
		OUT
		IN
		OUT
		IN
		OUT
		IN
		OUT
		IN
		OUT
		IN
		OUT
		IN
		OUT
		IN
		OUT

IV. DUPLICATE PROFICIENCY EVALUATION FORMS

STUDENT:		DATE:			
PROCEDURE (TASK): VITAL SIGNS					

SETTING: ☐ LABORATORY ☐ OTHER: (SPECIFY) ☐ CLINIC	SATISFACTORY	UNSATISFACTORY	NOT OBSERVED	NOT APPLICABLE
CONDITIONS (DESCRIBE)				
EQUIPMENT UTILIZED:				
STEPS IN PROCEDURE OR TASK:				
PATIENT PREPARATION				
1. Washes hands				
2. Checks chart (graphic history, vital signs)				
3. Identifies patient, self, and department				
4. Explains procedure and confirms patient understanding				
IMPLEMENTATION				
5. Positions patient (provides for privacy, comfort)				
6. Palpates appropriate artery				
7. Counts pulsations for specified time				
8. Notes rate, force, and rythmicity of beats				
9. Observes rate, depth, and rythmicity of respirations				
10. Repositions patient				
11. Reassures patient				
FOLLOW-UP				
12. Records pertinent data in chart and departmental records				
13. Notifies appropriate personnel				

STUDENT'S COMPREHENSION OF PROCEDURE (SELECT ONE ONLY)

The student demonstrates comprehensive knowledge of basic and advanced concepts beyond requirements of procedure	
The student demonstrates above average understanding of basic concepts applicable to the skill demonstrated	
The student demonstrates adequate knowledge of the essential elements of the task performed	
The student shows limited understanding of essential concepts related to the procedure	
The student has inadequate knowledge of even the basic concepts related to the task at hand	

OUTCOME CRITERIA (WHERE APPLICABLE)

☐ MET	SPECIFY CRITERIA NOT MET AND/OR PERTINENT CONSTRAINTS
☐ NOT MET	
☐ NOT APPL.	

ADDITIONAL COMMENTS

Include errors of omission or commission; if clinical therapeutic procedure emphasize communicative skills (verbal and non-verbal) and effectiveness of patient interaction:

SUMMARY PERFORMANCE EVALUATION AND RECOMMENDATIONS

SETTING	SATISFACTORY	UNSATISFACTORY	SPECIFY DEFICIENCIES
LABORATORY	☐ Can now perform skill under direct clinical super-vision	☐ Requires additional laboratory practice	
CLINIC	☐ Ready for min-imally supervised application and refinement	☐ Requires additional supervised clinical practice ☐ Complete re-evaluation required ☐ Re-evaluation·minor deficiencies only	

STUDENT: EVALUATOR: FACULTY:

STUDENT:	DATE:

PROCEDURE (TASK): ARTERIAL BLOOD PRESSURE

SETTING: ☐ LABORATORY ☐ OTHER: (SPECIFY) ☐ CLINIC	SATISFACTORY	UNSATISFACTORY	NOT OBSERVED	NOT APPLICABLE
CONDITIONS (DESCRIBE)				
EQUIPMENT UTILIZED:				

STEPS IN PROCEDURE OR TASK:				
EQUIPMENT AND PATIENT PREPARATION				
1. Washes hands				
2. Selects, gathers, and assembles appropriate equipment				
3. Checks chart (graphic history, vital signs, contraindications)				
4. Identifies patient, self, and department				
5. Explains procedure and confirms patient understanding				
IMPLEMENTATION				
6. Positions patient				
7. Positions/secures cuff properly				
8. Adjusts stethoscope position				
9. Closes pump valve				
10. Inflates cuff				
11. Reassures patient				
12. Opens valve, releases pressure slowly				
13. Observes manometer/listens to pulse sounds				
14. Records systolic/diasystolic pressures				
15. Repeats procedure to confirm results				
16. Removes equipment from patient's arm				
17. Reassures patient (repositions if necessary)				
FOLLOW-UP				
18. Records readings on appropriate records				
19. Maintains/processes equipment				
20. Notifies appropriate personnel				

STUDENT'S COMPREHENSION OF PROCEDURE (SELECT ONE ONLY)

The student demonstrates comprehensive knowledge of basic and advanced concepts beyond requirements of procedure	
The student demonstrates above average understanding of basic concepts applicable to the skill demonstrated	
The student demonstrates adequate knowledge of the essential elements of the task performed	
The student shows limited understanding of essential concepts related to the procedure	
The student has inadequate knowledge of even the basic concepts related to the task at hand	

OUTCOME CRITERIA (WHERE APPLICABLE)

☐ MET	SPECIFY CRITERIA NOT MET AND/OR PERTINENT CONSTRAINTS
☐ NOT MET	
☐ NOT APPL.	

ADDITIONAL COMMENTS

Include errors of omission or commission; if clinical therapeutic procedure emphasize communicative skills (verbal and non-verbal) and effectiveness of patient interaction:

SUMMARY PERFORMANCE EVALUATION AND RECOMMENDATIONS

SETTING	SATISFACTORY	UNSATISFACTORY	SPECIFY DEFICIENCIES
LABORATORY	☐ Can now perform skill under direct clinical supervision	☐ Requires additional laboratory practice	

CLINIC	☐ Ready for minimally supervised application and refinement	☐ Requires additional supervised clinical practice
		    ☐ Complete re-evaluation required
		    ☐ Re-evaluation·minor deficiencies only	

STUDENT: EVALUATOR: FACULTY:

STUDENT:	DATE:

PROCEDURE (TASK): PATIENT POSITIONING

SETTING: ☐ LABORATORY ☐ OTHER: (SPECIFY) ☐ CLINIC	SATISFACTORY	UNSATISFACTORY	NOT OBSERVED	NOT APPLICABLE
CONDITIONS (DESCRIBE)				
EQUIPMENT UTILIZED:				

STEPS IN PROCEDURE OR TASK:

EQUIPMENT AND PATIENT PREPARATION				
1. Washes hands				
2. Selects and gathers appropriate equipment				
3. Checks chart for order/contraindications to positioning				
4. Identifies patient, self, and department				
5. Explains procedure and confirms patient understanding				
IMPLEMENTATION				
6. Provides patient privacy				
7. Adjusts bed to working level				
8. Lowers siderails				
9. Removes supportive pillows				
10. Positions patient/bed				
11. Restores supportive aids				
12. Adjusts patient's body alignment				
13. Provides protection against pressure points				
14. Raises siderails				
FOLLOW-UP				
15. Provides for patient's safety/comfort				
16. Rechecks alignment/support of patient				
17. Repositions as necessary (steps 5-14 above)				
18. Records change of position and patient observations				
19. Notifies appropriate personnel				

STUDENT'S COMPREHENSION OF PROCEDURE (SELECT ONE ONLY)

The student demonstrates comprehensive knowledge of basic and advanced concepts beyond requirements of procedure	
The student demonstrates above average understanding of basic concepts applicable to the skill demonstrated	
The student demonstrates adequate knowledge of the essential elements of the task performed	
The student shows limited understanding of essential concepts related to the procedure	
The student has inadequate knowledge of even the basic concepts related to the task at hand	

OUTCOME CRITERIA (WHERE APPLICABLE)

☐ MET	SPECIFY CRITERIA NOT MET AND/OR PERTINENT CONSTRAINTS
☐ NOT MET	
☐ NOT APPL.	

ADDITIONAL COMMENTS

Include errors of omission or commission; if clinical therapeutic procedure emphasize communicative skills (verbal and non-verbal) and effectiveness of patient interaction:

SUMMARY PERFORMANCE EVALUATION AND RECOMMENDATIONS

SETTING	SATISFACTORY	UNSATISFACTORY	SPECIFY DEFICIENCIES
LABORATORY	☐ Can now perform skill under direct clinical super-vision	☐ Requires additional laboratory practice	

CLINIC	☐ Ready for min-imally supervised application and refinement	☐ Requires additional supervised clinical practice
		   ☐ Complete re-evaluation required
		   ☐ Re-evaluation·minor deficiencies only	

STUDENT: EVALUATOR: FACULTY:

STUDENT:	DATE:				

PROCEDURE (TASK): PATIENT ASSESSMENT					

	SATISFACTORY	UNSATISFACTORY	NOT OBSERVED	NOT APPLICABLE
SETTING: ☐ LABORATORY ☐ OTHER: (SPECIFY) ☐ CLINIC				
CONDITIONS (DESCRIBE)				
EQUIPMENT UTILIZED:				

STEPS IN PROCEDURE OR TASK:

	SATISFACTORY	UNSATISFACTORY	NOT OBSERVED	NOT APPLICABLE
EQUIPMENT AND PATIENT PREPARATION	▓	▓	▓	▓
1. Washes hands				
2. Selects, gathers, and assembles appropriate equipment				
3. Reviews pertinent chart information				
4. Identifies patient, self, and department				
5. Explains procedure and confirms patient understanding				
IMPLEMENTATION	▓	▓	▓	▓
6. Positions patient (provides for privacy, comfort)				
7. Assesses patient's vital signs				
8. Inspects patient's thorax				
9. Palpates patient's thorax				
10. Percusses patient's thorax				
11. Auscultates patient's thorax				
12. Measures patient's ventilatory parameters				
13. Repositions patient, clothing, bedding				
14. Reassures patient				
FOLLOW-UP	▓	▓	▓	▓
15. Maintains/processes equipment				
16. Records pertinent data in chart and departmental records				
17. Notifies appropriate personnel				

STUDENT'S COMPREHENSION OF PROCEDURE (SELECT ONE ONLY)

The student demonstrates comprehensive knowledge of basic and advanced concepts beyond requirements of procedure	
The student demonstrates above average understanding of basic concepts applicable to the skill demonstrated	
The student demonstrates adequate knowledge of the essential elements of the task performed	
The student shows limited understanding of essential concepts related to the procedure	
The student has inadequate knowledge of even the basic concepts related to the task at hand	

OUTCOME CRITERIA (WHERE APPLICABLE)

☐ MET	SPECIFY CRITERIA NOT MET AND/OR PERTINENT CONSTRAINTS
☐ NOT MET	
☐ NOT APPL.	

ADDITIONAL COMMENTS

Include errors of omission or commission; if clinical therapeutic procedure emphasize communicative skills (verbal and non-verbal) and effectiveness of patient interaction:

SUMMARY PERFORMANCE EVALUATION AND RECOMMENDATIONS

SETTING	SATISFACTORY	UNSATISFACTORY	SPECIFY DEFICIENCIES
LABORATORY	☐ Can now perform skill under direct clinical supervision	☐ Requires additional laboratory practice	

CLINIC	☐ Ready for minimally supervised application and refinement	☐ Requires additional supervised clinical practice
		  ☐ Complete re-evaluation required
		  ☐ Re-evaluation·minor deficiencies only	

STUDENT: EVALUATOR: FACULTY:

STUDENT:	DATE:

PROCEDURE (TASK): MEDICAL RECORDS

SETTING: ☐ LABORATORY ☐ OTHER: (SPECIFY) ☐ CLINIC	SATISFACTORY	UNSATISFACTORY	NOT OBSERVED	NOT APPLICABLE
CONDITIONS (DESCRIBE)				
EQUIPMENT UTILIZED:				

STEPS IN PROCEDURE OR TASK:				
IMPLEMENTATION				
1. Identifies and locates patient chart				
2. Informs appropriate personnel of chart use/location				
3. Ascertains and summarizes				
a. age/admitting diagnosis				
b. drug allergies				
c. current medications				
d. pertinent medical history/physical condition				
e. present condition				
f. diagnostic studies in progress				
4. Determines most current respiratory therapy orders				
5. Explains rationale for ordered therapy				
6. Evaluates appropriateness of respiratory therapy orders				
7. Suggests alternative therapy/rationale				
8. Implements therapy				
9. Records objective/subjective evaluation of patient response to therapy				
10. Explains ethical/legal principles of medical record-keeping				
FOLLOW-UP				
11. Returns chart to proper location				
12. Informs appropriate personnel				

STUDENT'S COMPREHENSION OF PROCEDURE (SELECT ONE ONLY)

The student demonstrates comprehensive knowledge of basic and advanced concepts beyond requirements of procedure	
The student demonstrates above average understanding of basic concepts applicable to the skill demonstrated	
The student demonstrates adequate knowledge of the essential elements of the task performed	
The student shows limited understanding of essential concepts related to the procedure	
The student has inadequate knowledge of even the basic concepts related to the task at hand	

OUTCOME CRITERIA (WHERE APPLICABLE)

☐ MET	SPECIFY CRITERIA NOT MET AND/OR PERTINENT CONSTRAINTS
☐ NOT MET	
☐ NOT APPL.	

ADDITIONAL COMMENTS

Include errors of omission or commission; if clinical therapeutic procedure emphasize communicative skills (verbal and non-verbal) and effectiveness of patient interaction:

SUMMARY PERFORMANCE EVALUATION AND RECOMMENDATIONS

SETTING	SATISFACTORY	UNSATISFACTORY	SPECIFY DEFICIENCIES
LABORATORY	☐ Can now perform skill under direct clinical supervision	☐ Requires additional laboratory practice	
CLINIC	☐ Ready for minimally supervised application and refinement	☐ Requires additional supervised clinical practice 　☐ Complete re-evaluation required 　☐ Re-evaluation·minor deficiencies only	

STUDENT:　　　　　　EVALUATOR:　　　　　FACULTY:

STUDENT:		DATE:

PROCEDURE (TASK): HANDWASHING

	SATISFACTORY	UNSATISFACTORY	NOT OBSERVED	NOT APPLICABLE
SETTING: ☐ LABORATORY ☐ OTHER: (SPECIFY) ☐ CLINIC				
CONDITIONS (DESCRIBE)				
EQUIPMENT UTILIZED:				

STEPS IN PROCEDURE OR TASK:

	SATISFACTORY	UNSATISFACTORY	NOT OBSERVED	NOT APPLICABLE
PREPARATION				
1. Removes jewelry				
2. Prevents clothing contact with sink				
3. Turns water on (warm)				
IMPLEMENTATION				
4. Wets hands				
5. Applies soap/disinfectant thoroughly				
6. Washes palms/back of hands with rotary motion (20 sec.)				
7. Washes fingers/spaces with interlacing motion (10 sec.)				
8. Washes wrists and above (4 in.) with rotary motion				
9. Repeats steps 5 through 8				
10. Rinses well from wrists to fingers				
11. Dries with aseptic towel				
FOLLOW-UP				
12. Turns off water aseptically				
13. Discards materials in receptacle				
14. Repeats procedure if contaminated				

STUDENT'S COMPREHENSION OF PROCEDURE (SELECT ONE ONLY)

The student demonstrates comprehensive knowledge of basic and advanced concepts beyond requirements of procedure	
The student demonstrates above average understanding of basic concepts applicable to the skill demonstrated	
The student demonstrates adequate knowledge of the essential elements of the task performed	
The student shows limited understanding of essential concepts related to the procedure	
The student has inadequate knowledge of even the basic concepts related to the task at hand	

OUTCOME CRITERIA (WHERE APPLICABLE)

☐ MET	SPECIFY CRITERIA NOT MET AND/OR PERTINENT CONSTRAINTS
☐ NOT MET	
☐ NOT APPL.	

ADDITIONAL COMMENTS

Include errors of omission or commission; if clinical therapeutic procedure emphasize communicative skills (verbal and non-verbal) and effectiveness of patient interaction:

SUMMARY PERFORMANCE EVALUATION AND RECOMMENDATIONS

SETTING	SATISFACTORY	UNSATISFACTORY	SPECIFY DEFICIENCIES
LABORATORY	☐ Can now perform skill under direct clinical super-vision	☐ Requires additional laboratory practice	
CLINIC	☐ Ready for min-imally supervised application and refinement	☐ Requires additional supervised clinical practice ☐ Complete re-evaluation required ☐ Re-evaluation·minor deficiencies only	

STUDENT: EVALUATOR: FACULTY:

STUDENT:		DATE:				

PROCEDURE (TASK): CHEMICAL DISINFECTION AND STERILIZATION

	SATISFACTORY	UNSATISFACTORY	NOT OBSERVED	NOT APPLICABLE
SETTING: ☐ LABORATORY ☐ OTHER: (SPECIFY) ☐ CLINIC				
CONDITIONS (DESCRIBE)				
EQUIPMENT UTILIZED:				

STEPS IN PROCEDURE OR TASK:

	SATISFACTORY	UNSATISFACTORY	NOT OBSERVED	NOT APPLICABLE
EQUIPMENT PROCUREMENT AND PREPARATION	▨	▨	▨	▨
1. Isolates, gathers and transports equipment to site				
2. Disinfects sinks (washer)				
3. Fills wash sink, adds detergent				
4. Sorts, disassembles equipment				
5. Immerses and scrubs equipment (institutes wash cycle)				
6. Rinses equipment (institutes rinse cycle)				
7. Drains equipment				
DISINFECTION/STERILIZATION	▨	▨	▨	▨
8. Checks solution expiration date				
9. Immerses equipment in solution (institutes disinfection cycle)				
10. Soaks equipment for specified interval				
11. Drains and rinses equipment (institutes rinse cycle)				
12. Dries equipment (institutes spin dry cycle)				
FOLLOW-UP	▨	▨	▨	▨
13. Washes hands				
14. Reassembles equipment				
15. Cultures equipment sample(s)				
16. Bags, seals, labels, dates equipment				
17. Stores equipment, rotates stock				

STUDENT'S COMPREHENSION OF PROCEDURE (SELECT ONE ONLY)

The student demonstrates comprehensive knowledge of basic and advanced concepts beyond requirements of procedure	
The student demonstrates above average understanding of basic concepts applicable to the skill demonstrated	
The student demonstrates adequate knowledge of the essential elements of the task performed	
The student shows limited understanding of essential concepts related to the procedure	
The student has inadequate knowledge of even the basic concepts related to the task at hand	

OUTCOME CRITERIA (WHERE APPLICABLE)

☐ MET	SPECIFY CRITERIA NOT MET AND/OR PERTINENT CONSTRAINTS
☐ NOT MET	
☐ NOT APPL.	

ADDITIONAL COMMENTS

Include errors of omission or commission; if clinical therapeutic procedure emphasize communicative skills (verbal and non-verbal) and effectiveness of patient interaction:

SUMMARY PERFORMANCE EVALUATION AND RECOMMENDATIONS

SETTING	SATISFACTORY	UNSATISFACTORY	SPECIFY DEFICIENCIES
LABORATORY	☐ Can now perform skill under direct clinical super-vision	☐ Requires additional laboratory practice	
CLINIC	☐ Ready for min-imally supervised application and refinement	☐ Requires additional supervised clinical practice ☐ Complete re-evaluation required ☐ Re-evaluation·minor deficiencies only	

STUDENT: EVALUATOR: FACULTY:

STUDENT:		DATE:				

PROCEDURE (TASK): GAS STERILIZATION

SETTING: ☐ LABORATORY ☐ OTHER: (SPECIFY) ☐ CLINIC						

STEPS IN PROCEDURE OR TASK:	SATISFACTORY	UNSATISFACTORY	NOT OBSERVED	NOT APPLICABLE
CONDITIONS (DESCRIBE)				
EQUIPMENT UTILIZED:				
EQUIPMENT PROCUREMENT AND PREPARATION	▓	▓	▓	▓
1. Isolates, gathers, and transports equipment to site				
2. Disinfects sinks (washer)				
3. Fills wash sink, adds detergent				
4. Sorts, disassembles equipment				
5. Immerses and scrubs equipment (institutes wash cycle)				
6. Rinses equipment (institutes rinse cycle)				
7. Dries equipment				
8. Washes hands				
9. Reassembles equipment				
10. Bags, seals, labels, dates equipment				
STERILIZATION	▓	▓	▓	▓
11. Inserts equipment in sterilizer with indicator				
12. Runs and logs sterilization cycle				
FOLLOW-UP	▓	▓	▓	▓
13. Aerates equipment				
14. Incubates test indicator				
15. Verifies sterility				
16. Stores equipment, rotates stock				

STUDENT'S COMPREHENSION OF PROCEDURE (SELECT ONE ONLY)

The student demonstrates comprehensive knowledge of basic and advanced concepts beyond requirements of procedure	
The student demonstrates above average understanding of basic concepts applicable to the skill demonstrated	
The student demonstrates adequate knowledge of the essential elements of the task performed	
The student shows limited understanding of essential concepts related to the procedure	
The student has inadequate knowledge of even the basic concepts related to the task at hand	

OUTCOME CRITERIA (WHERE APPLICABLE)

☐ MET	SPECIFY CRITERIA NOT MET AND/OR PERTINENT CONSTRAINTS
☐ NOT MET	
☐ NOT APPL.	

ADDITIONAL COMMENTS

Include errors of omission or commission; if clinical therapeutic procedure emphasize communicative skills (verbal and non-verbal) and effectiveness of patient interaction:

SUMMARY PERFORMANCE EVALUATION AND RECOMMENDATIONS

SETTING	SATISFACTORY	UNSATISFACTORY	SPECIFY DEFICIENCIES
LABORATORY	☐ Can now perform skill under direct clinical supervision	☐ Requires additional laboratory practice	
CLINIC	☐ Ready for minimally supervised application and refinement	☐ Requires additional supervised clinical practice ☐ Complete re-evaluation required ☐ Re-evaluation·minor deficiencies only	

STUDENT: EVALUATOR: FACULTY:

STUDENT:				DATE:			

PROCEDURE (TASK): PASTEURIZATION

	SATISFACTORY	UNSATISFACTORY	NOT OBSERVED	NOT APPLICABLE
SETTING: ☐ LABORATORY ☐ OTHER: (SPECIFY) ☐ CLINIC				
CONDITIONS (DESCRIBE)				
EQUIPMENT UTILIZED:				

STEPS IN PROCEDURE OR TASK:

	SATISFACTORY	UNSATISFACTORY	NOT OBSERVED	NOT APPLICABLE
EQUIPMENT PROCUREMENT AND PREPARATION				
1. Isolates, gathers, and transports equipment to site				
2. Disinfects sink (washer)				
3. Fills wash sink, adds detergent				
4. Sorts, disassembles equipment				
5. Immerses and scrubs equipment (institutes wash cycle)				
6. Rinses equipment (institutes rinse cycle)				
7. Drains equipment				
PASTEURIZATION				
8. Confirms water bath temperature				
9. Immerses equipment in water bath				
10. Soaks equipment for specified interval				
11. Drains equipment				
12. Dries equipment				
FOLLOW-UP				
13. Washes hands				
14. Reassembles equipment				
15. Cultures equipment sample(s)				
16. Bags, seals, labels, dates equipment				
17. Stores equipment, rotates stock				

STUDENT'S COMPREHENSION OF PROCEDURE (SELECT ONE ONLY)

The student demonstrates comprehensive knowledge of basic and advanced concepts beyond requirements of procedure	
The student demonstrates above average understanding of basic concepts applicable to the skill demonstrated	
The student demonstrates adequate knowledge of the essential elements of the task performed	
The student shows limited understanding of essential concepts related to the procedure	
The student has inadequate knowledge of even the basic concepts related to the task at hand	

OUTCOME CRITERIA (WHERE APPLICABLE)

☐ MET	SPECIFY CRITERIA NOT MET AND/OR PERTINENT CONSTRAINTS
☐ NOT MET	
☐ NOT APPL.	

ADDITIONAL COMMENTS

Include errors of omission or commission; if clinical therapeutic procedure emphasize communicative skills (verbal and non-verbal) and effectiveness of patient interaction:

SUMMARY PERFORMANCE EVALUATION AND RECOMMENDATIONS

SETTING	SATISFACTORY	UNSATISFACTORY	SPECIFY DEFICIENCIES
LABORATORY	☐ Can now perform skill under direct clinical supervision	☐ Requires additional laboratory practice	
CLINIC	☐ Ready for minimally supervised application and refinement	☐ Requires additional supervised clinical practice ☐ Complete re-evaluation required ☐ Re-evaluation·minor deficiencies only	

STUDENT: EVALUATOR: FACULTY:

STUDENT:	DATE:				

PROCEDURE (TASK): BACTERIOLOGICAL SURVEILLANCE

SETTING: ☐ LABORATORY ☐ OTHER: (SPECIFY) ☐ CLINIC	SATISFACTORY	UNSATISFACTORY	NOT OBSERVED	NOT APPLICABLE
CONDITIONS (DESCRIBE)				
EQUIPMENT UTILIZED:				

STEPS IN PROCEDURE OR TASK:				
EQUIPMENT PREPARATION				
1. Selects and gathers appropriate equipment				
2. Checks (ensures) sterility of sampling and transfer apparatus				
3. Washes hands				
4. Opens sampling (culture transfer) packaging				
SAMPLING PROCEDURE				
5. Selects appropriate location/technique for obtaining sample				
6. Obtain adequate sample aseptically				
7. Labels, logs sample as to equipment, location, status, date				
8. Isolates sample				
9. Transfers sample to culture/growth media				
10. Incubates sample (delivers to laboratory)				
FOLLOW-UP				
11. Monitors culture media for bacteriological growth (secures lab report				
12. Evaluates presence/nature of bacteriological growth (lab report)				
13. Takes appropriate action				
14. Maintains records/results of actions taken				

STUDENT'S COMPREHENSION OF PROCEDURE (SELECT ONE ONLY)

The student demonstrates comprehensive knowledge of basic and advanced concepts beyond requirements of procedure	
The student demonstrates above average understanding of basic concepts applicable to the skill demonstrated	
The student demonstrates adequate knowledge of the essential elements of the task performed	
The student shows limited understanding of essential concepts related to the procedure	
The student has inadequate knowledge of even the basic concepts related to the task at hand	

OUTCOME CRITERIA (WHERE APPLICABLE)

☐ MET	SPECIFY CRITERIA NOT MET AND/OR PERTINENT CONSTRAINTS
☐ NOT MET	
☐ NOT APPL.	

ADDITIONAL COMMENTS

Include errors of omission or commission; if clinical therapeutic procedure emphasize communicative skills (verbal and non-verbal) and effectiveness of patient interaction:

SUMMARY PERFORMANCE EVALUATION AND RECOMMENDATIONS

SETTING	SATISFACTORY	UNSATISFACTORY	SPECIFY DEFICIENCIES
LABORATORY	☐ Can now perform skill under direct clinical super-vision	☐ Requires additional laboratory practice	
CLINIC	☐ Ready for min-imally supervised application and refinement	☐ Requires additional supervised clinical practice ☐ Complete re-evaluation required ☐ Re-evaluation·minor deficiencies only	

STUDENT: EVALUATOR: FACULTY:

STUDENT:	DATE:				

PROCEDURE (TASK): ISOLATION					

SETTING: ☐ LABORATORY ☐ OTHER: (SPECIFY) ☐ CLINIC	SATISFACTORY	UNSATISFACTORY	NOT OBSERVED	NOT APPLICABLE
CONDITIONS (DESCRIBE)				
EQUIPMENT UTILIZED:				

STEPS IN PROCEDURE OR TASK:				
PREPARATION				
1. Verifies type, nature and purpose of isolation				
2. Washes hands				
3. Selects and gathers appropriate equipment				
IMPLEMENTATION				
4. Dons protective shoe/hair coverings				
5. Dons, closes, and fastens gown				
6. Applies mask				
7. Dons gloves over gown				
8. Enters room, explains procedure to patient				
9. Performs duties, reassures patient				
10. Discards contaminated supplies				
11. Bags, seals, labels, and transfers contaminated equipment				
12. Removes, discards shoe coverings, gloves				
13. Unfastens gown				
14. Removes, discards gown, mask, haircovering				
FOLLOW-UP				
15. Washes hands				
16. Maintains/processes equipment				
17. Records pertinent data in chart and departmental records				
18. Notifies appropriate personnel				

STUDENT'S COMPREHENSION OF PROCEDURE (SELECT ONE ONLY)

The student demonstrates comprehensive knowledge of basic and advanced concepts beyond requirements of procedure	
The student demonstrates above average understanding of basic concepts applicable to the skill demonstrated	
The student demonstrates adequate knowledge of the essential elements of the task performed	
The student shows limited understanding of essential concepts related to the procedure	
The student has inadequate knowledge of even the basic concepts related to the task at hand	

OUTCOME CRITERIA (WHERE APPLICABLE)

☐ MET	SPECIFY CRITERIA NOT MET AND/OR PERTINENT CONSTRAINTS
☐ NOT MET	
☐ NOT APPL.	

ADDITIONAL COMMENTS

Include errors of omission or commission; if clinical therapeutic procedure emphasize communicative skills (verbal and non-verbal) and effectiveness of patient interaction:

SUMMARY PERFORMANCE EVALUATION AND RECOMMENDATIONS

SETTING	SATISFACTORY	UNSATISFACTORY	SPECIFY DEFICIENCIES
LABORATORY	☐ Can now perform skill under direct clinical supervision	☐ Requires additional laboratory practice	
CLINIC	☐ Ready for minimally supervised application and refinement	☐ Requires additional supervised clinical practice ☐ Complete re-evaluation required ☐ Re-evaluation·minor deficiencies only	

STUDENT: EVALUATOR: FACULTY:

STUDENT:	DATE:				

PROCEDURE (TASK): CYLINDER SAFETY AND TRANSPORT					

		SATISFACTORY	UNSATISFACTORY	NOT OBSERVED	NOT APPLICABLE
SETTING: ☐ LABORATORY ☐ OTHER: (SPECIFY) ☐ CLINIC					
CONDITIONS (DESCRIBE)					
EQUIPMENT UTILIZED:					

STEPS IN PROCEDURE OR TASK:		SATISFACTORY	UNSATISFACTORY	NOT OBSERVED	NOT APPLICABLE
EQUIPMENT PREPARATION					
1.	Selects appropriate cylinder (size, content)				
2.	Maneuvers cylinder properly to cart or stand				
3.	Secures cylinder				
4.	Removes valve stem cap or cover				
5.	Cracks cylinder				
IMPLEMENTATION					
6.	Selects appropriate regulator				
7.	Attaches regulator to cylinder valve stem				
8.	Slowly opens cylinder valve				
9.	Checks regulator/cylinder assembly for leakage/fit				
10.	Reads cylinder contents				
11.	Estimates duration of flow for specified use				
12.	Transports cylinder properly to destination				
13.	Connects specified equipment to regulator				
14.	Follows oxygen safety precautions (where applicable)				
FOLLOW-UP					
15.	Schedules cylinder content check/change at correct time				
16.	If gas not in use, turns cylinder valve off, evacuates regulator				

STUDENT'S COMPREHENSION OF PROCEDURE (SELECT ONE ONLY)

The student demonstrates comprehensive knowledge of basic and advanced concepts beyond requirements of procedure	
The student demonstrates above average understanding of basic concepts applicable to the skill demonstrated	
The student demonstrates adequate knowledge of the essential elements of the task performed	
The student shows limited understanding of essential concepts related to the procedure	
The student has inadequate knowledge of even the basic concepts related to the task at hand	

OUTCOME CRITERIA (WHERE APPLICABLE)

☐ MET	SPECIFY CRITERIA NOT MET AND/OR PERTINENT CONSTRAINTS
☐ NOT MET	
☐ NOT APPL.	

ADDITIONAL COMMENTS

Include errors of omission or commission; if clinical therapeutic procedure emphasize communicative skills (verbal and non-verbal) and effectiveness of patient interaction:

SUMMARY PERFORMANCE EVALUATION AND RECOMMENDATIONS

SETTING	SATISFACTORY	UNSATISFACTORY	SPECIFY DEFICIENCIES
LABORATORY	☐ Can now perform skill under direct clinical supervision	☐ Requires additional laboratory practice	
CLINIC	☐ Ready for minimally supervised application and refinement	☐ Requires additional supervised clinical practice ☐ Complete re-evaluation required ☐ Re-evaluation·minor deficiencies only	

STUDENT:　　　　　EVALUATOR:　　　　　FACULTY:

358

STUDENT:	DATE:				

PROCEDURE (TASK): OXYGEN THERAPY

SETTING: ☐ LABORATORY ☐ OTHER: (SPECIFY) ☐ CLINIC		SATISFACTORY	UNSATISFACTORY	NOT OBSERVED	NOT APPLICABLE
CONDITIONS (DESCRIBE)					
EQUIPMENT UTILIZED:					

STEPS IN PROCEDURE OR TASK:	SATISFACTORY	UNSATISFACTORY	NOT OBSERVED	NOT APPLICABLE
EQUIPMENT AND PATIENT PREPARATION				
1. Washes hands				
2. Selects, gathers, and assembles appropriate equipment				
3. Verifies, interprets, and evaluates physician's order				
4. Identifies patient, self, and department				
5. Explains procedure and confirms patient understanding				
IMPLEMENTATION AND ASSESSMENT				
6. Adds sterile (distilled) water to humidifier/aerosol generator				
7. Connects humidifier (aerosol generator), flowmeter, oxygen modality				
8. Initiates gas flow				
9. Tests equipment for proper function				
10. Assesses patient (objective and subjective)				
11. Applies modality to patient, ensuring maximum comfort/safety				
12. Adjusts gas flow (oxygen concentration) appropriate to orders/objectives				
13. Assesses patient's response (objective and subjective)				
14. Modifies procedure to accommodate patient's response				
15. Analyzes F_IO_2 (where appropriate/feasible)				
16. Follows oxygen safety precautions (provides instructions to patient)				
FOLLOW-UP				
17. Maintains proper equipment function				
18. Records pertinent data in chart and department records				
19. Notifies appropriate personnel				

STUDENT'S COMPREHENSION OF PROCEDURE (SELECT ONE ONLY)

The student demonstrates comprehensive knowledge of basic and advanced concepts beyond requirements of procedure	
The student demonstrates above average understanding of basic concepts applicable to the skill demonstrated	
The student demonstrates adequate knowledge of the essential elements of the task performed	
The student shows limited understanding of essential concepts related to the procedure	
The student has inadequate knowledge of even the basic concepts related to the task at hand	

OUTCOME CRITERIA (WHERE APPLICABLE)

☐ MET	SPECIFY CRITERIA NOT MET AND/OR PERTINENT CONSTRAINTS
☐ NOT MET	
☐ NOT APPL.	

ADDITIONAL COMMENTS

Include errors of omission or commission; if clinical therapeutic procedure emphasize communicative skills (verbal and non-verbal) and effectiveness of patient interaction:

SUMMARY PERFORMANCE EVALUATION AND RECOMMENDATIONS

SETTING	SATISFACTORY	UNSATISFACTORY	SPECIFY DEFICIENCIES
LABORATORY	☐ Can now perform skill under direct clinical super-vision	☐ Requires additional laboratory practice	
CLINIC	☐ Ready for min-imally supervised application and refinement	☐ Requires additional supervised clinical practice ☐ Complete re-evaluation required ☐ Re-evaluation·minor deficiencies only	

STUDENT: EVALUATOR: FACULTY:

STUDENT:		DATE:				

PROCEDURE (TASK): OXYHOOD

SETTING: ☐ LABORATORY ☐ OTHER: (SPECIFY) ☐ CLINIC	SATISFACTORY	UNSATISFACTORY	NOT OBSERVED	NOT APPLICABLE
CONDITIONS (DESCRIBE)				
EQUIPMENT UTILIZED:				

STEPS IN PROCEDURE OR TASK:

	SATISFACTORY	UNSATISFACTORY	NOT OBSERVED	NOT APPLICABLE
EQUIPMENT AND PATIENT PREPARATION	▨	▨	▨	▨
1. Washes hands				
2. Selects, gathers, and assembles appropriate equipment				
3. Verifies, interprets, and evaluates physician's orders				
4. Explains procedures to parents and confirms understanding				
IMPLEMENTATION AND ASSESSMENT	▨	▨	▨	▨
5. Properly fills humidifier or nebulizer with sterile, distilled water				
6. Attaches humidifier or nebulizer to appropriate gas sources				
7. Preheats humidifier/nebulizer				
8. Connects tubing to enclosure				
9. Initiates proper gas flowrate/checks for proper function				
10. Places infant in enclosure/ensures proper fit and patient comfort				
11. Analyzes F_1O_2 and ensures proper level				
12. Monitors temperature and ensures proper level				
13. Monitors and assesses patient's status/obtains objective/subjective data on oxygenation				
14. Readjust therapy as indicated				
15. Provides for continuous (if applicable) temperature and F_1O_2 monitoring				
FOLLOW-UP	▨	▨	▨	▨
16. Maintains/processes equipment				
17. Records pertinent data in chart and department records				
18. Notifies appropriate personnel				

STUDENT'S COMPREHENSION OF PROCEDURE (SELECT ONE ONLY)

The student demonstrates comprehensive knowledge of basic and advanced concepts beyond requirements of procedure	
The student demonstrates above average understanding of basic concepts applicable to the skill demonstrated	
The student demonstrates adequate knowledge of the essential elements of the task performed	
The student shows limited understanding of essential concepts related to the procedure	
The student has inadequate knowledge of even the basic concepts related to the task at hand	

OUTCOME CRITERIA (WHERE APPLICABLE)

☐ MET	SPECIFY CRITERIA NOT MET AND/OR PERTINENT CONSTRAINTS
☐ NOT MET	
☐ NOT APPL.	

ADDITIONAL COMMENTS

Include errors of omission or commission; if clinical therapeutic procedure emphasize communicative skills (verbal and non-verbal) and effectiveness of patient interaction:

SUMMARY PERFORMANCE EVALUATION AND RECOMMENDATIONS

SETTING	SATISFACTORY	UNSATISFACTORY	SPECIFY DEFICIENCIES
LABORATORY	☐ Can now perform skill under direct clinical supervision	☐ Requires additional laboratory practice	

CLINIC	☐ Ready for minimally supervised application and refinement	☐ Requires additional supervised clinical practice
		  ☐ Complete re-evaluation required
		  ☐ Re-evaluation·minor deficiencies only	

STUDENT: EVALUATOR: FACULTY:

STUDENT:		DATE:				

PROCEDURE (TASK): MEASUREMENT OF OXYGEN CONCENTRATIONS

SETTING: ☐ LABORATORY ☐ OTHER: (SPECIFY) ☐ CLINIC	SATISFACTORY	UNSATISFACTORY	NOT OBSERVED	NOT APPLICABLE
CONDITIONS (DESCRIBE)				
EQUIPMENT UTILIZED:				

STEPS IN PROCEDURE OR TASK:

	SATISFACTORY	UNSATISFACTORY	NOT OBSERVED	NOT APPLICABLE
EQUIPMENT AND PATIENT PREPARATION	▓	▓	▓	▓
1. Selects and gathers appropriate analyzer, accessories				
2. Verifies physician's order for specified F_IO_2				
3. Identifies patient, self, department				
4. Explains procedure and confirms patient understanding				
IMPLEMENTATION	▓	▓	▓	▓
5. Checks for proper electrical function of analyzer				
6. Check dessicant or balast (where applicable)				
7. Calibrates analyzer on room air (balance)				
8. Slopes analyzer to 100% O_2 or specific known concentration				
9. Places probe (sampling tube) in gas atmosphere				
10. Takes sample or waits for full response				
11. Makes reading				
12. Corrects for temperature, humidity or pressure (where applicable)				
13. Removes or secures probe/sampling tube				
14. Turns analyzer off				
FOLLOW-UP	▓	▓	▓	▓
15. Records oxygen concentration in appropriate records				
16. Maintains equipment				
17. Notifies appropriate personnel				
18. Rechecks oxygen concentration as required				

STUDENT'S COMPREHENSION OF PROCEDURE (SELECT ONE ONLY)

The student demonstrates comprehensive knowledge of basic and advanced concepts beyond requirements of procedure	
The student demonstrates above average understanding of basic concepts applicable to the skill demonstrated	
The student demonstrates adequate knowledge of the essential elements of the task performed	
The student shows limited understanding of essential concepts related to the procedure	
The student has inadequate knowledge of even the basic concepts related to the task at hand	

OUTCOME CRITERIA (WHERE APPLICABLE)

☐ MET	SPECIFY CRITERIA NOT MET AND/OR PERTINENT CONSTRAINTS
☐ NOT MET	
☐ NOT APPL.	

ADDITIONAL COMMENTS

Include errors of omission or commission; if clinical therapeutic procedure emphasize communicative skills (verbal and non-verbal) and effectiveness of patient interaction:

SUMMARY PERFORMANCE EVALUATION AND RECOMMENDATIONS

SETTING	SATISFACTORY	UNSATISFACTORY	SPECIFY DEFICIENCIES
LABORATORY	☐ Can now perform skill under direct clinical supervision	☐ Requires additional laboratory practice	
CLINIC	☐ Ready for minimally supervised application and refinement	☐ Requires additional supervised clinical practice ☐ Complete re-evaluation required ☐ Re-evaluation·minor deficiencies only	

STUDENT: EVALUATOR: FACULTY:

STUDENT:	DATE:

PROCEDURE (TASK): AEROSOL/HUMIDITY THERAPY

SETTING: ☐ LABORATORY ☐ OTHER: (SPECIFY)
          ☐ CLINIC

CONDITIONS (DESCRIBE)

EQUIPMENT UTILIZED:

STEPS IN PROCEDURE OR TASK:

	SATISFACTORY	UNSATISFACTORY	NOT OBSERVED	NOT APPLICABLE
EQUIPMENT AND PATIENT PREPARATION				
1. Washes hands				
2. Selects, gathers, and assembles appropriate equipment				
3. Verifies, interprets, and evaluates physician's order				
4. Identifies patient, self, and department				
5. Explains procedure and confirms patient understanding				
IMPLEMENTATION AND ASSESSMENT				
6. Adds appropriate solution aseptically and in correct amount				
7. Connects humidifier/aerosol generator to appropriate gas source				
8. Initiates gas flow/aerosol generation				
9. Tests equipment for proper function				
10. Applies modality to patient, ensuring maximum comfort/safety				
11. Ensures gas flow and oxygen concentration appropriate to order/ objectives				
12. Adjusts humidity (aerosol output), temperature appropriate to order/ objectives				
13. Gives additional instructions, where necessary, to maximize therapeutic benefit				
14. Assesses patient response (subjective/objective)				
15. Modifies technique to deal with adverse response				
FOLLOW-UP				
16. Maintains proper equipment function				
17. Records pertinent data in chart and department records				
18. Notifies appropriate personnel				

STUDENT'S COMPREHENSION OF PROCEDURE (SELECT ONE ONLY)

The student demonstrates comprehensive knowledge of basic and advanced concepts beyond requirements of procedure	
The student demonstrates above average understanding of basic concepts applicable to the skill demonstrated	
The student demonstrates adequate knowledge of the essential elements of the task performed	
The student shows limited understanding of essential concepts related to the procedure	
The student has inadequate knowledge of even the basic concepts related to the task at hand	

OUTCOME CRITERIA (WHERE APPLICABLE)

☐ MET	SPECIFY CRITERIA NOT MET AND/OR PERTINENT CONSTRAINTS
☐ NOT MET	
☐ NOT APPL.	

ADDITIONAL COMMENTS

Include errors of omission or commission; if clinical therapeutic procedure emphasize communicative skills (verbal and non-verbal) and effectiveness of patient interaction:

SUMMARY PERFORMANCE EVALUATION AND RECOMMENDATIONS

SETTING	SATISFACTORY	UNSATISFACTORY	SPECIFY DEFICIENCIES
LABORATORY	☐ Can now perform skill under direct clinical super-vision	☐ Requires additional laboratory practice	
CLINIC	☐ Ready for min-imally supervised application and refinement	☐ Requires additional supervised clinical practice ☐ Complete re-evaluation required ☐ Re-evaluation·minor deficiencies only	

STUDENT: EVALUATOR: FACULTY:

STUDENT:		DATE:				

PROCEDURE (TASK): AEROSOL ENCLOSURES					

SETTING: ☐ LABORATORY ☐ OTHER: (SPECIFY) ☐ CLINIC	SATISFACTORY	UNSATISFACTORY	NOT OBSERVED	NOT APPLICABLE
CONDITIONS (DESCRIBE)				
EQUIPMENT UTILIZED:				

STEPS IN PROCEDURE OR TASK:

	SATISFACTORY	UNSATISFACTORY	NOT OBSERVED	NOT APPLICABLE
EQUIPMENT AND PATIENT PREPARATION				
1. Washes hands				
2. Selects, gathers, and assembles appropriate equipment				
3. Verifies, interprets, and evaluates physician's order				
4. Identifies patient, self, and department				
5. Explains procedure and confirms patient (family) understanding				
IMPLEMENTATION AND ASSESSMENT				
6. Attaches canopy to frame and secures to bed (crib)				
7. Connects aerosol generator to appropriate gas source				
8. Adds appropriate solution aseptically in correct amount				
9. Tests equipment for proper function				
10. Initiates gas flow and fills enclosure with aerosol				
11. Introduces patient into enclosure				
12. Adjusts gas flow, aerosol output and temperature appropriate to objectives				
13. Ensures patient comfort, canopy fit				
14. Measures F_IO_2, adjusts to prescribed level				
15. Assesses patient response (objective and subjective)				
16. Modifies technique to accommodate response				
17. Follows oxygen safety precautions				
FOLLOW-UP				
18. Maintains proper equipment function				
19. Records pertinent data in chart and department records				
20. Notifies appropriate personnel				

STUDENT'S COMPREHENSION OF PROCEDURE (SELECT ONE ONLY)

The student demonstrates comprehensive knowledge of basic and advanced concepts beyond requirements of procedure	
The student demonstrates above average understanding of basic concepts applicable to the skill demonstrated	
The student demonstrates adequate knowledge of the essential elements of the task performed	
The student shows limited understanding of essential concepts related to the procedure	
The student has inadequate knowledge of even the basic concepts related to the task at hand	

OUTCOME CRITERIA (WHERE APPLICABLE)

☐ MET	SPECIFY CRITERIA NOT MET AND/OR PERTINENT CONSTRAINTS
☐ NOT MET	
☐ NOT APPL.	

ADDITIONAL COMMENTS

Include errors of omission or commission; if clinical therapeutic procedure emphasize communicative skills (verbal and non-verbal) and effectiveness of patient interaction:

SUMMARY PERFORMANCE EVALUATION AND RECOMMENDATIONS

SETTING	SATISFACTORY	UNSATISFACTORY	SPECIFY DEFICIENCIES
LABORATORY	☐ Can now perform skill under direct clinical supervision	☐ Requires additional laboratory practice	
CLINIC	☐ Ready for minimally supervised application and refinement	☐ Requires additional supervised clinical practice ☐ Complete re-evaluation required ☐ Re-evaluation·minor deficiencies only	

STUDENT: EVALUATOR: FACULTY:

STUDENT:		DATE:				

PROCEDURE (TASK): AEROSOL DRUG ADMINISTRATION

	SATISFACTORY	UNSATISFACTORY	NOT OBSERVED	NOT APPLICABLE
SETTING: ☐ LABORATORY ☐ OTHER: (SPECIFY) ☐ CLINIC				
CONDITIONS (DESCRIBE)				
EQUIPMENT UTILIZED:				

STEPS IN PROCEDURE OR TASK:

	SATISFACTORY	UNSATISFACTORY	NOT OBSERVED	NOT APPLICABLE
EQUIPMENT AND PATIENT PREPARATION				
1. Washes hands				
2. Selects, gathers, and assembles appropriate equipment				
3. Verifies, interprets, and evaluates physician's order				
4. Identifies patient, self, and department				
5. Explains procedure and confirms patient understanding				
IMPLEMENTATION AND ASSESSMENT				
6. Pre-assesses patient (objective and subjective) to establish baseline values				
7. Connects aerosol generator to appropriate gas source				
8. Determines and measures proper dosage of drug/diluent				
9. Adds prescribed drug/diluent to nebulizer chamber				
10. Initiates gas flow				
11. Test equipment for proper function				
12. Properly positions patient				
13. Applies modality to patient, ensuring maximum comfort/safety				
14. Encourages and ensures proper breathing pattern				
15. Adjust gas flow/aerosol output to maximize therapeutic benefit				
16. Checks patient's vital signs, observes response				
17. Modifies technique to deal with adverse patient response				
18. Terminates therapy when complete dosage administered				
19. Encourages patient cough, collects, examines sputum				
20. Conducts post-assessment (objective and subjective), compares to initial measures				
FOLLOW-UP				
21. Maintains/processes equipment				
22. Records pertinent data in chart and department records				
23. Notifies appropriate personnel				

STUDENT'S COMPREHENSION OF PROCEDURE (SELECT ONE ONLY)

The student demonstrates comprehensive knowledge of basic and advanced concepts beyond requirements of procedure	
The student demonstrates above average understanding of basic concepts applicable to the skill demonstrated	
The student demonstrates adequate knowledge of the essential elements of the task performed	
The student shows limited understanding of essential concepts related to the procedure	
The student has inadequate knowledge of even the basic concepts related to the task at hand	

OUTCOME CRITERIA (WHERE APPLICABLE)

☐ MET	SPECIFY CRITERIA NOT MET AND/OR PERTINENT CONSTRAINTS
☐ NOT MET	
☐ NOT APPL.	

ADDITIONAL COMMENTS

Include errors of omission or commission; if clinical therapeutic procedure emphasize communicative skills (verbal and non-verbal) and effectiveness of patient interaction:

SUMMARY PERFORMANCE EVALUATION AND RECOMMENDATIONS

SETTING	SATISFACTORY	UNSATISFACTORY	SPECIFY DEFICIENCIES
LABORATORY	☐ Can now perform skill under direct clinical supervision	☐ Requires additional laboratory practice	

CLINIC	☐ Ready for minimally supervised application and refinement	☐ Requires additional supervised clinical practice
		  ☐ Complete re-evaluation required
		  ☐ Re-evaluation·minor deficiencies only	

STUDENT: EVALUATOR: FACULTY:

STUDENT:	DATE:				

PROCEDURE (TASK): INCENTIVE SPIROMETRY

	SATISFACTORY	UNSATISFACTORY	NOT OBSERVED	NOT APPLICABLE
SETTING: ☐ LABORATORY ☐ OTHER: (SPECIFY) ☐ CLINIC				
CONDITIONS (DESCRIBE)				
EQUIPMENT UTILIZED:				

STEPS IN PROCEDURE OR TASK:

EQUIPMENT AND PATIENT PREPARATION				
1. Washes hands				
2. Selects, gathers, and assembles appropriate equipment				
3. Verifies, interprets, and evaluates physician's order				
4. Identifies patient, self, and department				
5. Explains procedure and confirms patient understanding				
IMPLEMENTATION AND ASSESSMENT				
6. Tests equipment for proper function				
7. Positions patient (and spirometer) properly				
8. Determines patient's inspiratory capacity				
9. Sets appropriate initial goal				
10. Institutes therapy, encourages patient's maximum effort				
11. Observes and evaluates patient response				
12. Readjusts goal appropriate to patient response				
13. Terminates therapy when goal/repetitions achieved				
FOLLOW-UP				
14. Provides instructions to patient on independent use of device				
15. Records pertinent data (progress) in chart and department records				
16. Maintains/processes equipment				
17. Notifies appropriate personnel				

STUDENT'S COMPREHENSION OF PROCEDURE (SELECT ONE ONLY)

The student demonstrates comprehensive knowledge of basic and advanced concepts beyond requirements of procedure	
The student demonstrates above average understanding of basic concepts applicable to the skill demonstrated	
The student demonstrates adequate knowledge of the essential elements of the task performed	
The student shows limited understanding of essential concepts related to the procedure	
The student has inadequate knowledge of even the basic concepts related to the task at hand	

OUTCOME CRITERIA (WHERE APPLICABLE)

☐ MET	SPECIFY CRITERIA NOT MET AND/OR PERTINENT CONSTRAINTS
☐ NOT MET	
☐ NOT APPL.	

ADDITIONAL COMMENTS

Include errors of omission or commission; if clinical therapeutic procedure emphasize communicative skills (verbal and non-verbal) and effectiveness of patient interaction:

SUMMARY PERFORMANCE EVALUATION AND RECOMMENDATIONS

SETTING	SATISFACTORY	UNSATISFACTORY	SPECIFY DEFICIENCIES
LABORATORY	☐ Can now perform skill under direct clinical supervision	☐ Requires additional laboratory practice	

CLINIC	☐ Ready for minimally supervised application and refinement	☐ Requires additional supervised clinical practice
		   ☐ Complete re-evaluation required
		   ☐ Re-evaluation·minor deficiencies only	

STUDENT: EVALUATOR: FACULTY:

STUDENT:	DATE:				

PROCEDURE (TASK): INTERMITTENT POSITIVE PRESSURE BREATHING

SETTING: ☐ LABORATORY ☐ OTHER: (SPECIFY) ☐ CLINIC	SATISFACTORY	UNSATISFACTORY	NOT OBSERVED	NOT APPLICABLE
CONDITIONS (DESCRIBE)				
EQUIPMENT UTILIZED:				

STEPS IN PROCEDURE OR TASK:

	SATISFACTORY	UNSATISFACTORY	NOT OBSERVED	NOT APPLICABLE
EQUIPMENT AND PATIENT PREPARATION	▨	▨	▨	▨
1. Washes hands				
2. Selects, gathers, and assembles appropriate equipment				
3. Verifies, interprets, and evaluates physician's order				
4. Identifies patient, self, and department				
5. Explains procedure and confirms patient understanding				
IMPLEMENTATION AND ASSESSMENT	▨	▨	▨	▨
6. Connects breathing circuit to ventilator				
7. Provides power (pneumatic/electrical) to ventilator				
8. Measures proper dosage of drug/diluent, adds to nebulizer				
9. Cycles ventilator, tests for proper function				
10. Sets initial ventilator values appropriate for patient				
11. Properly positions patient				
12. Pre-assesses patient (objective and subjective)				
13. Applies breathing circuit to patient's airway, initiates therapy				
14. Instructs patient, adjusts ventilator to maintain appropriate parameters				
15. Observes patient response				
16. Modifies technique to accommodate patient's response				
17. Reassesses patient's vital signs, ventilatory parameters				
18. Terminates procedure after appropriate interval				
19. Encourages patient cough, collects, examines sputum				
20. Conducts post-assessment (objective and subjective)				
FOLLOW-UP	▨	▨	▨	▨
21. Maintains/processes equipment				
22. Records pertinent data in chart and department records				
23. Notifies appropriate personnel				

STUDENT'S COMPREHENSION OF PROCEDURE (SELECT ONE ONLY)

The student demonstrates comprehensive knowledge of basic and advanced concepts beyond requirements of procedure	
The student demonstrates above average understanding of basic concepts applicable to the skill demonstrated	
The student demonstrates adequate knowledge of the essential elements of the task performed	
The student shows limited understanding of essential concepts related to the procedure	
The student has inadequate knowledge of even the basic concepts related to the task at hand	

OUTCOME CRITERIA (WHERE APPLICABLE)

☐ MET	SPECIFY CRITERIA NOT MET AND/OR PERTINENT CONSTRAINTS
☐ NOT MET	
☐ NOT APPL.	

ADDITIONAL COMMENTS

Include errors of omission or commission; if clinical therapeutic procedure emphasize communicative skills (verbal and non-verbal) and effectiveness of patient interaction:

SUMMARY PERFORMANCE EVALUATION AND RECOMMENDATIONS

SETTING	SATISFACTORY	UNSATISFACTORY	SPECIFY DEFICIENCIES
LABORATORY	☐ Can now perform skill under direct clinical super-vision	☐ Requires additional laboratory practice	
CLINIC	☐ Ready for min-imally supervised application and refinement	☐ Requires additional supervised clinical practice ☐ Complete re-evaluation required ☐ Re-evaluation·minor deficiencies only	

STUDENT: EVALUATOR: FACULTY:

STUDENT:		DATE:				

PROCEDURE (TASK): BREATHING EXERCISES

SETTING: ☐ LABORATORY ☐ OTHER: (SPECIFY)
☐ CLINIC

CONDITIONS (DESCRIBE)

EQUIPMENT UTILIZED:

STEPS IN PROCEDURE OR TASK:	SATISFACTORY	UNSATISFACTORY	NOT OBSERVED	NOT APPLICABLE
EQUIPMENT AND PATIENT PREPARATION				
1. Washes hands				
2. Selects, gathers, and assembles appropriate equipment				
3. Verifies, interprets, and evaluates physician's order				
4. Identifies patient, self, and department				
5. Explains procedure and confirms patient understanding				
IMPLEMENTATION AND ASSESSMENT				
6. Positions patient				
7. Demonstrates procedure on self				
8. Observes/palpates applicable muscle activity				
9. Instructs patient to coordinate applicable muscle activity				
10. Applies inspiratory resistance to applicable muscle group				
11. Encourages slow, forceful inspiration, passive exhalation				
12. Observes and corrects common errors				
13. Repeats procedure as indicated/tolerated				
FOLLOW-UP				
14. Demonstrates methods of self-application				
15. Provides reinforcement for conformance				
16. Returns patient to comfortable position				
17. Records pertinent data in chart and departmental records				
18. Maintains/processes equipment				
19. Notifies appropriate personnel				

STUDENT'S COMPREHENSION OF PROCEDURE (SELECT ONE ONLY)

The student demonstrates comprehensive knowledge of basic and advanced concepts beyond requirements of procedure	
The student demonstrates above average understanding of basic concepts applicable to the skill demonstrated	
The student demonstrates adequate knowledge of the essential elements of the task performed	
The student shows limited understanding of essential concepts related to the procedure	
The student has inadequate knowledge of even the basic concepts related to the task at hand	

OUTCOME CRITERIA (WHERE APPLICABLE)

☐ MET	SPECIFY CRITERIA NOT MET AND/OR PERTINENT CONSTRAINTS
☐ NOT MET	
☐ NOT APPL.	

ADDITIONAL COMMENTS

Include errors of omission or commission; if clinical therapeutic procedure emphasize communicative skills (verbal and non-verbal) and effectiveness of patient interaction:

SUMMARY PERFORMANCE EVALUATION AND RECOMMENDATIONS

SETTING	SATISFACTORY	UNSATISFACTORY	SPECIFY DEFICIENCIES
LABORATORY	☐ Can now perform skill under direct clinical supervision	☐ Requires additional laboratory practice	
CLINIC	☐ Ready for minimally supervised application and refinement	☐ Requires additional supervised clinical practice ☐ Complete re-evaluation required ☐ Re-evaluation·minor deficiencies only	

STUDENT: EVALUATOR: FACULTY:

STUDENT:		DATE:			

PROCEDURE (TASK): COUGHING

	SATISFACTORY	UNSATISFACTORY	NOT OBSERVED	NOT APPLICABLE
SETTING: ☐ LABORATORY ☐ OTHER: (SPECIFY) ☐ CLINIC				
CONDITIONS (DESCRIBE)				
EQUIPMENT UTILIZED:				

STEPS IN PROCEDURE OR TASK:

EQUIPMENT AND PATIENT PREPARATION				
1. Washes hands				
2. Selects, gathers, and assembles appropriate equipment				
3. Verifies, interprets, and evaluates physician's order				
4. Identifies patient, self, and department				
5. Explains procedure and confirms patient understanding				
IMPLEMENTATION AND ASSESSMENT				
6. Positions patient				
7. Pre-assesses patient				
8. Instructs patient in effective use of diaphragm				
9. Demonstrates cough phases on self				
10. Provides incisional support (postoperative)				
11. Encourages deep inspiration, inspiratory hold				
12. Assures forceful contraction of abdominal muscles				
13. Observes and corrects common errors				
14. Modifies technique as appropriate to patient				
15. Reassesses patient				
16. Repeats procedure as indicated/tolerated				
17. Examines (collects) sputum				
FOLLOW-UP				
18. Provides reinforcement for conformance				
19. Returns patient to comfortable position				
20. Records pertinent data in chart and department records				
21. Maintains/processes equipment				
22. Notifies appropriate personnel				

STUDENT'S COMPREHENSION OF PROCEDURE (SELECT ONE ONLY)

The student demonstrates comprehensive knowledge of basic and advanced concepts beyond requirements of procedure	
The student demonstrates above average understanding of basic concepts applicable to the skill demonstrated	
The student demonstrates adequate knowledge of the essential elements of the task performed	
The student shows limited understanding of essential concepts related to the procedure	
The student has inadequate knowledge of even the basic concepts related to the task at hand	

OUTCOME CRITERIA (WHERE APPLICABLE)

	SPECIFY CRITERIA NOT MET AND/OR PERTINENT CONSTRAINTS
☐ MET	
☐ NOT MET	
☐ NOT APPL.	

ADDITIONAL COMMENTS

Include errors of omission or commission; if clinical therapeutic procedure emphasize communicative skills (verbal and non-verbal) and effectiveness of patient interaction:

SUMMARY PERFORMANCE EVALUATION AND RECOMMENDATIONS

SETTING	SATISFACTORY	UNSATISFACTORY	SPECIFY DEFICIENCIES
LABORATORY	☐ Can now perform skill under direct clinical super-vision	☐ Requires additional laboratory practice	
CLINIC	☐ Ready for min-imally supervised application and refinement	☐ Requires additional supervised clinical practice ☐ Complete re-evaluation required ☐ Re-evaluation·minor deficiencies only	

STUDENT: EVALUATOR: FACULTY:

STUDENT:	DATE:

PROCEDURE (TASK): POSTURAL DRAINAGE AND PERCUSSION

SETTING: ☐ LABORATORY ☐ OTHER: (SPECIFY) ☐ CLINIC CONDITIONS (DESCRIBE) EQUIPMENT UTILIZED:	SATISFACTORY	UNSATISFACTORY	NOT OBSERVED	NOT APPLICABLE
STEPS IN PROCEDURE OR TASK:				
EQUIPMENT AND PATIENT PREPARATION				
1. Washes hands				
2. Selects, gathers, and assembles appropriate equipment				
3. Verifies, interprets, and evaluates physician's order				
4. Identifies patient, self, and department				
5. Explains procedure and confirms patient understanding				
IMPLEMENTATION AND ASSESSMENT				
6. Pre-assesses patient				
7. Instructs (demonstrates) patient in diaphragmatic breathing, segmental expansion and coughing				
8. Positions patient for segmental/lobar drainage				
9. Assesses patient response/tolerance				
10. Modifies position to accommodate patient's response				
11. Encourages maintenance of proper breathing pattern				
12. Performs percussion over properly identified area				
13. Perform vibration over correct area during expiration				
14. Encourages and assists patient with cough/expectoration				
15. Examines (collects) sputum				
16. Maintains position for appropriate time interval				
17. Repositions patient and repeats procedure as indicated/tolerated				
18. Returns patient to comfortable position				
19. Reassesses patient				
FOLLOW-UP				
20. Provides reinforcement for conformance				
21. Records pertinent data in chart and department records				
22. Maintains/processes equipment				
23. Notifies appropriate personnel				

STUDENT'S COMPREHENSION OF PROCEDURE (SELECT ONE ONLY)

The student demonstrates comprehensive knowledge of basic and advanced concepts beyond requirements of procedure	
The student demonstrates above average understanding of basic concepts applicable to the skill demonstrated	
The student demonstrates adequate knowledge of the essential elements of the task performed	
The student shows limited understanding of essential concepts related to the procedure	
The student has inadequate knowledge of even the basic concepts related to the task at hand	

OUTCOME CRITERIA (WHERE APPLICABLE)

☐ MET	SPECIFY CRITERIA NOT MET AND/OR PERTINENT CONSTRAINTS
☐ NOT MET	
☐ NOT APPL.	

ADDITIONAL COMMENTS

Include errors of omission or commission; if clinical therapeutic procedure emphasize communicative skills (verbal and non-verbal) and effectiveness of patient interaction:

SUMMARY PERFORMANCE EVALUATION AND RECOMMENDATIONS

SETTING	SATISFACTORY	UNSATISFACTORY	SPECIFY DEFICIENCIES
LABORATORY	☐ Can now perform skill under direct clinical supervision	☐ Requires additional laboratory practice	
CLINIC	☐ Ready for minimally supervised application and refinement	☐ Requires additional supervised clinical practice ☐ Complete re-evaluation required ☐ Re-evaluation·minor deficiencies only	

STUDENT: EVALUATOR: FACULTY:

STUDENT:	DATE:				

PROCEDURE (TASK): CARDIOPULMONARY RESUSCITATION (ADULT)

SETTING: ☐ LABORATORY ☐ OTHER: (SPECIFY) ☐ CLINIC	SATISFACTORY	UNSATISFACTORY	NOT OBSERVED	NOT APPLICABLE
CONDITIONS (DESCRIBE)				
EQUIPMENT UTILIZED:				

STEPS IN PROCEDURE OR TASK:				
ASSESSMENT				
1. Establishes unresponsiveness				
2. Summons help				
3. Opens airway/establishes breathlessness				
4. Identifies arrhythmia (if monitored)				
IMPLEMENTATION (BASIC LIFE SUPPORT)				
5. Administers four quick breaths				
6. Clears airway (obstruction)				
7. Establishes pulselessness				
8. Initiates chest compressions/maintains ventilation				
9. Checks for return of pulse and spontaneous breathing				
10. Maintains effective ventilation/compression ratio				
IMPLEMENTATION (ADVANCED LIFE SUPPORT)				
11. Selects, inserts and secures airway adjunct				
12. Selects and applies manual ventilator (oxygenates)				
13. Checks for return of pulse and spontaneous breathing				
14. Aspirates airway				
15. Continues support as indicated				
FOLLOW-UP				
16. Provides post-resuscitative support/care				
17. Maintains/processes equipment				
18. Records pertinent data in chart and departmental records				

STUDENT'S COMPREHENSION OF PROCEDURE (SELECT ONE ONLY)

The student demonstrates comprehensive knowledge of basic and advanced concepts beyond requirements of procedure	
The student demonstrates above average understanding of basic concepts applicable to the skill demonstrated	
The student demonstrates adequate knowledge of the essential elements of the task performed	
The student shows limited understanding of essential concepts related to the procedure	
The student has inadequate knowledge of even the basic concepts related to the task at hand	

OUTCOME CRITERIA (WHERE APPLICABLE)

☐ MET	SPECIFY CRITERIA NOT MET AND/OR PERTINENT CONSTRAINTS
☐ NOT MET	
☐ NOT APPL.	

ADDITIONAL COMMENTS

Include errors of omission or commission; if clinical therapeutic procedure emphasize communicative skills (verbal and non-verbal) and effectiveness of patient interaction:

SUMMARY PERFORMANCE EVALUATION AND RECOMMENDATIONS

SETTING	SATISFACTORY	UNSATISFACTORY	SPECIFY DEFICIENCIES
LABORATORY	☐ Can now perform skill under direct clinical supervision	☐ Requires additional laboratory practice	
CLINIC	☐ Ready for minimally supervised application and refinement	☐ Requires additional supervised clinical practice ☐ Complete re-evaluation required ☐ Re-evaluation·minor deficiencies only	

STUDENT: EVALUATOR: FACULTY:

STUDENT:	DATE:				

PROCEDURE (TASK):CARDIOPULMONARY RESUSCITATION (Infant/Child)					

SETTING: ☐ LABORATORY ☐ OTHER: (SPECIFY) ☐ CLINIC	SATISFACTORY	UNSATISFACTORY	NOT OBSERVED	NOT APPLICABLE
CONDITIONS (DESCRIBE)				
EQUIPMENT UTILIZED:				

STEPS IN PROCEDURE OR TASK:				
ASSESSMENT	▒	▒	▒	▒
1. Establishes unresponsiveness				
2. Summons help				
3. Opens airway/establishes breathlessness				
4. Identifies arrhythmia (if monitored)				
IMPLEMENTATION (BASIC LIFE SUPPORT)	▒	▒	▒	▒
5. Administers four quick breaths				
6. Clears airway (obstruction)				
7. Establishes pulselessness				
8. Initiates chest compressions/maintains ventilation				
9. Checks for return of pulse and spontaneous breathing				
10. Maintains effective ventilation/compression ratio				
IMPLEMENTATION (ADVANCED LIFE SUPPORT)	▒	▒	▒	▒
11. Selects, inserts, and secures airway adjunct				
12. Selects and applies manual ventilator (oxygenates)				
13. Checks for return of pulse and spontaneous breathing				
14. Aspirates airway				
15. Continues support as indicated				
FOLLOW-UP	▒	▒	▒	▒
16. Provides post-resuscitative support/care				
17. Maintains/processes equipment				
18. Records pertinent data in chart and departmental records				

STUDENT'S COMPREHENSION OF PROCEDURE (SELECT ONE ONLY)

The student demonstrates comprehensive knowledge of basic and advanced concepts beyond requirements of procedure	
The student demonstrates above average understanding of basic concepts applicable to the skill demonstrated	
The student demonstrates adequate knowledge of the essential elements of the task performed	
The student shows limited understanding of essential concepts related to the procedure	
The student has inadequate knowledge of even the basic concepts related to the task at hand	

OUTCOME CRITERIA (WHERE APPLICABLE)

☐ MET	SPECIFY CRITERIA NOT MET AND/OR PERTINENT CONSTRAINTS
☐ NOT MET	
☐ NOT APPL.	

ADDITIONAL COMMENTS

Include errors of omission or commission; if clinical therapeutic procedure emphasize communicative skills (verbal and non-verbal) and effectiveness of patient interaction:

SUMMARY PERFORMANCE EVALUATION AND RECOMMENDATIONS

SETTING	SATISFACTORY	UNSATISFACTORY	SPECIFY DEFICIENCIES
LABORATORY	☐ Can now perform skill under direct clinical super-vision	☐ Requires additional laboratory practice	
CLINIC	☐ Ready for min-imally supervised application and refinement	☐ Requires additional supervised clinical practice ☐ Complete re-evaluation required ☐ Re-evaluation·minor deficiencies only	

STUDENT: EVALUATOR: FACULTY:

STUDENT:		DATE:		

PROCEDURE (TASK): EMERGENCY ENDOTRACHEAL INTUBATION

SETTING: ☐ LABORATORY ☐ OTHER: (SPECIFY)
          ☐ CLINIC

CONDITIONS (DESCRIBE)

EQUIPMENT UTILIZED:

STEPS IN PROCEDURE OR TASK:

	SATISFACTORY	UNSATISFACTORY	NOT OBSERVED	NOT APPLICABLE
EQUIPMENT AND PATIENT PREPARATION				
1. Washes hands				
2. Selects, gathers, and assembles appropriate equipment				
3. Explains procedure and confirms patient understanding				
4. Provides for sedation (where necessary)				
IMPLEMENTATION				
5. Positions patient				
6. Clears airway				
7. Anesthetizes airway				
8. Hyperoxygenates patient				
9. Inserts laryngoscope into oropharynx				
10. Exposes, lifts epiglottis and visualizes cords				
11. Inserts endotracheal tube through vocal cords				
12. Inflates tube cuff				
13. Provides ventilation, hyperoxygenation				
14. Auscultates chest for symmetrical ventilation				
FOLLOW-UP				
15. Marks proximal end of tube				
16. Secures and stabilizes tube				
17. Aspirates trachea, bronchi				
18. Provides post-intubation care/support				
19. Provides for follow-up chest radiograph				
20. Maintains/processes equipment				
21. Records pertinent data in chart and departmental records				
22. Notifies appropriate personnel				

STUDENT'S COMPREHENSION OF PROCEDURE (SELECT ONE ONLY)

The student demonstrates comprehensive knowledge of basic and advanced concepts beyond requirements of procedure	
The student demonstrates above average understanding of basic concepts applicable to the skill demonstrated	
The student demonstrates adequate knowledge of the essential elements of the task performed	
The student shows limited understanding of essential concepts related to the procedure	
The student has inadequate knowledge of even the basic concepts related to the task at hand	

OUTCOME CRITERIA (WHERE APPLICABLE)

☐ MET	SPECIFY CRITERIA NOT MET AND/OR PERTINENT CONSTRAINTS
☐ NOT MET	
☐ NOT APPL.	

ADDITIONAL COMMENTS

Include errors of omission or commission; if clinical therapeutic procedure emphasize communicative skills (verbal and non-verbal) and effectiveness of patient interaction:

SUMMARY PERFORMANCE EVALUATION AND RECOMMENDATIONS

SETTING	SATISFACTORY	UNSATISFACTORY	SPECIFY DEFICIENCIES
LABORATORY	☐ Can now perform skill under direct clinical supervision	☐ Requires additional laboratory practice	
CLINIC	☐ Ready for minimally supervised application and refinement	☐ Requires additional supervised clinical practice ☐ Complete re-evaluation required ☐ Re-evaluation·minor deficiencies only	

STUDENT: EVALUATOR: FACULTY:

STUDENT:		DATE:				

PROCEDURE (TASK): TRACHEOBRONCHIAL ASPIRATION					

	SATISFACTORY	UNSATISFACTORY	NOT OBSERVED	NOT APPLICABLE
SETTING: ☐ LABORATORY ☐ OTHER: (SPECIFY) ☐ CLINIC				
CONDITIONS (DESCRIBE)				
EQUIPMENT UTILIZED:				

STEPS IN PROCEDURE OR TASK:				
EQUIPMENT AND PATIENT PREPARATION				
1. Selects, gathers, and assembles appropriate equipment				
2. Identifies patient, self, and department				
3. Explains procedure and confirms patient understanding				
IMPLEMENTATION AND ASSESSMENT				
4. Assesses patient/patient airway				
5. Hyperoxygenates and hyperinflates patient				
6. Washes hands				
7. Adjusts suction to appropriate level				
8. Positions patient				
9. Dons sterile glove(s)				
10. Pours (sterile) water into (sterile) bowl				
11. Attaches sputum trap to suction source				
12. Attaches catheter to suction source				
13. Reassures patient				
14. Inserts catheter until resistance met				
15. Withdraws catheter 1 to 2 centimeters				
16. Applies intermittent suction, rotates/withdraws catheter				
17. Clears catheter, repeats as necessary				
18. Hyperoxygenates and hyperinflates patient				
19. Reassesses patient/patient airway				
20. Reassures patient				
FOLLOW-UP				
21. Restores patient to prior status				
22. Maintains/processes equipment				
23. Records pertinent data in chart and departmental records				
24. Notifies appropriate personnel				

STUDENT'S COMPREHENSION OF PROCEDURE (SELECT ONE ONLY)

The student demonstrates comprehensive knowledge of basic and advanced concepts beyond requirements of procedure	
The student demonstrates above average understanding of basic concepts applicable to the skill demonstrated	
The student demonstrates adequate knowledge of the essential elements of the task performed	
The student shows limited understanding of essential concepts related to the procedure	
The student has inadequate knowledge of even the basic concepts related to the task at hand	

OUTCOME CRITERIA (WHERE APPLICABLE)

☐ MET	SPECIFY CRITERIA NOT MET AND/OR PERTINENT CONSTRAINTS
☐ NOT MET	
☐ NOT APPL.	

ADDITIONAL COMMENTS

Include errors of omission or commission; if clinical therapeutic procedure emphasize communicative skills (verbal and non-verbal) and effectiveness of patient interaction:

SUMMARY PERFORMANCE EVALUATION AND RECOMMENDATIONS

SETTING	SATISFACTORY	UNSATISFACTORY	SPECIFY DEFICIENCIES
LABORATORY	☐ Can now perform skill under direct clinical super-vision	☐ Requires additional laboratory practice	

CLINIC	☐ Ready for min-imally supervised application and refinement	☐ Requires additional supervised clinical practice
		  ☐ Complete re-evaluation required
		  ☐ Re-evaluation·minor deficiencies only	

STUDENT:　　　　　EVALUATOR:　　　　FACULTY:

STUDENT:		DATE:			

PROCEDURE (TASK): CUFF MANAGEMENT					

SETTING: ☐ LABORATORY ☐ OTHER: (SPECIFY) ☐ CLINIC	SATISFACTORY	UNSATISFACTORY	NOT OBSERVED	NOT APPLICABLE
CONDITIONS (DESCRIBE)				
EQUIPMENT UTILIZED:				

STEPS IN PROCEDURE OR TASK:	SATISFACTORY	UNSATISFACTORY	NOT OBSERVED	NOT APPLICABLE
EQUIPMENT AND PATIENT PREPARATION	▨	▨	▨	▨
1. Washes hands				
2. Selects, gathers, and assembles appropriate equipment				
3. Verifies, interprets, and evaluates physician's order				
4. Identifies patient, self, and department				
5. Explains procedure and confirms patient's understanding				
IMPLEMENTATION	▨	▨	▨	▨
6. Aspirates oro/hypopharynx				
7. Deflates cuff				
8. Connects pressure gauge to cuff inflation line				
9. Connects syringe to "Y" fitting				
10. Provides inspiratory positive pressure				
11. Auscultates over cuff site				
12. Inflates cuff to minimal occluding volume				
13. Deflate cuff until minimal leak, observes pressure				
14. Secures cuff inflation inlet (valve)				
15. Reassures patient				
FOLLOW-UP	▨	▨	▨	▨
16. Maintains/processes equipment				
17. Records pertinent data in chart and departmental records				
18. Notifies appropriate personnel				

STUDENT'S COMPREHENSION OF PROCEDURE (SELECT ONE ONLY)

The student demonstrates comprehensive knowledge of basic and advanced concepts beyond requirements of procedure	
The student demonstrates above average understanding of basic concepts applicable to the skill demonstrated	
The student demonstrates adequate knowledge of the essential elements of the task performed	
The student shows limited understanding of essential concepts related to the procedure	
The student has inadequate knowledge of even the basic concepts related to the task at hand	

OUTCOME CRITERIA (WHERE APPLICABLE)

	SPECIFY CRITERIA NOT MET AND/OR PERTINENT CONSTRAINTS
☐ MET	
☐ NOT MET	
☐ NOT APPL.	

ADDITIONAL COMMENTS

Include errors of omission or commission; if clinical therapeutic procedure emphasize communicative skills (verbal and non-verbal) and effectiveness of patient interaction:

SUMMARY PERFORMANCE EVALUATION AND RECOMMENDATIONS

SETTING	SATISFACTORY	UNSATISFACTORY	SPECIFY DEFICIENCIES
LABORATORY	☐ Can now perform skill under direct clinical supervision	☐ Requires additional laboratory practice	
CLINIC	☐ Ready for minimally supervised application and refinement	☐ Requires additional supervised clinical practice ☐ Complete re-evaluation required ☐ Re-evaluation·minor deficiencies only	

STUDENT:　　　　　　　　EVALUATOR:　　　　　　　FACULTY:

STUDENT:	DATE:

PROCEDURE (TASK): TRACHEOSTOMY CARE

SETTING: ☐ LABORATORY ☐ OTHER: (SPECIFY)
☐ CLINIC

CONDITIONS (DESCRIBE)

EQUIPMENT UTILIZED:

STEPS IN PROCEDURE OR TASK:	SATISFACTORY	UNSATISFACTORY	NOT OBSERVED	NOT APPLICABLE
EQUIPMENT AND PATIENT PREPARATION				
1. Selects, gathers, and assembles appropriate equipment				
2. Verifies, interprets, and evaluates physician's order				
3. Identifies patient, self, and department				
4. Explains procedure and confirms patient understanding				
IMPLEMENTATION AND ASSESSMENT				
5. Positions patient				
6. Washes hands				
7. Dons sterile gloves				
8. Removes ties, stoma dressing				
9. Cleans stoma				
10. Removes inner cannula, cleans/rinses				
11. Replaces inner cannula, stabilizes				
12. Places new sterile dressing around tube				
13. Resecures tube with clean ties				
14. Rechecks tube position/stability				
15. Auscultates chest/cuff site				
16. Reassures patient				
FOLLOW-UP				
17. Restores patient to prior status				
18. Maintains/processes equipment				
19. Records pertinent data in chart and departmental records				
20. Notifies appropriate personnel				

STUDENT'S COMPREHENSION OF PROCEDURE (SELECT ONE ONLY)

The student demonstrates comprehensive knowledge of basic and advanced concepts beyond requirements of procedure	
The student demonstrates above average understanding of basic concepts applicable to the skill demonstrated	
The student demonstrates adequate knowledge of the essential elements of the task performed	
The student shows limited understanding of essential concepts related to the procedure	
The student has inadequate knowledge of even the basic concepts related to the task at hand	

OUTCOME CRITERIA (WHERE APPLICABLE)

☐ MET	SPECIFY CRITERIA NOT MET AND/OR PERTINENT CONSTRAINTS
☐ NOT MET	
☐ NOT APPL.	

ADDITIONAL COMMENTS

Include errors of omission or commission; if clinical therapeutic procedure emphasize communicative skills (verbal and non-verbal) and effectiveness of patient interaction:

SUMMARY PERFORMANCE EVALUATION AND RECOMMENDATIONS

SETTING	SATISFACTORY	UNSATISFACTORY	SPECIFY DEFICIENCIES
LABORATORY	☐ Can now perform skill under direct clinical supervision	☐ Requires additional laboratory practice	
CLINIC	☐ Ready for minimally supervised application and refinement	☐ Requires additional supervised clinical practice ☐ Complete re-evaluation required ☐ Re-evaluation·minor deficiencies only	

STUDENT: EVALUATOR: FACULTY:

STUDENT:	DATE:				

PROCEDURE (TASK): ENDOTRACHEAL EXTUBATION

	SATISFACTORY	UNSATISFACTORY	NOT OBSERVED	NOT APPLICABLE
SETTING: ☐ LABORATORY ☐ OTHER: (SPECIFY) ☐ CLINIC				
CONDITIONS (DESCRIBE)				
EQUIPMENT UTILIZED:				

STEPS IN PROCEDURE OR TASK:

	SATISFACTORY	UNSATISFACTORY	NOT OBSERVED	NOT APPLICABLE
EQUIPMENT AND PATIENT PREPARATION				
1. Selects, gathers, and assembles appropriate equipment				
2. Verifies, interprets, and evaluates physician's order				
3. Identifies patient, self, and department				
4. Explains procedure and confirms patient understanding				
IMPLEMENTATION AND ASSESSMENT				
5. Confirms ventilatory status/airway function				
6. Positions patient				
7. Aspirates trachea, oro/hypopharynx				
8. Hyperoxygenates and hyperinflates patient				
9. Unsecures tube				
10. Deflates cuff				
11. Passes suction catheter beyond tube tip				
12. Instructs patient to breath deeply				
13. Remove tube/catheter while applying suction				
14. Encourages patient to cough				
15. Reassures patient				
FOLLOW-UP				
16. Provides appropriate humidification and oxygenation				
17. Monitors and observes patient response				
18. Maintains/processes equipment				
19. Records pertinent data in chart and departmental record				
20. Notifies appropriate personnel				

STUDENT'S COMPREHENSION OF PROCEDURE (SELECT ONE ONLY)

The student demonstrates comprehensive knowledge of basic and advanced concepts beyond requirements of procedure	
The student demonstrates above average understanding of basic concepts applicable to the skill demonstrated	
The student demonstrates adequate knowledge of the essential elements of the task performed	
The student shows limited understanding of essential concepts related to the procedure	
The student has inadequate knowledge of even the basic concepts related to the task at hand	

OUTCOME CRITERIA (WHERE APPLICABLE)

☐ MET	SPECIFY CRITERIA NOT MET AND/OR PERTINENT CONSTRAINTS
☐ NOT MET	
☐ NOT APPL.	

ADDITIONAL COMMENTS

Include errors of omission or commission; if clinical therapeutic procedure emphasize communicative skills (verbal and non-verbal) and effectiveness of patient interaction:

SUMMARY PERFORMANCE EVALUATION AND RECOMMENDATIONS

SETTING	SATISFACTORY	UNSATISFACTORY	SPECIFY DEFICIENCIES
LABORATORY	☐ Can now perform skill under direct clinical supervision	☐ Requires additional laboratory practice	
CLINIC	☐ Ready for minimally supervised application and refinement	☐ Requires additional supervised clinical practice ☐ Complete re-evaluation required ☐ Re-evaluation·minor deficiencies only	

STUDENT: EVALUATOR: FACULTY:

STUDENT:		DATE:				

PROCEDURE (TASK): BEDSIDE VENTILATORY ASSESSMENT

SETTING: ☐ LABORATORY ☐ OTHER: (SPECIFY) ☐ CLINIC	SATISFACTORY	UNSATISFACTORY	NOT OBSERVED	NOT APPLICABLE
CONDITIONS (DESCRIBE)				
EQUIPMENT UTILIZED:				

STEPS IN PROCEDURE OR TASK:				
EQUIPMENT AND PATIENT PREPARATION				
1. Washes hands				
2. Selects, gathers, and assembles appropriate equipment				
3. Verifies, interprets, and evaluates physician's order				
4. Identifies patient, self, and department				
5. Explains procedure and confirms patient understanding				
IMPLEMENTATION AND ASSESSMENT				
6. Ensures ventilatory activity, checks airway				
7. Connects volumeter to airway				
8. Reassures patient				
9. Measures minute ventilation/observes response				
10. Restores patient to prior status				
11. Explains, demonstrates forced vital capacity maneuver				
12. Connects volumeter to airway				
13. Encourages/elicits maximum inspiration/forced expiration				
14. Repeats procedure for best patient effort				
15. Restores patient to prior status; reassures patient				
16. Explains, demonstrates inspiratory force maneuver				
17. Connect manometer/valve assembly to airway				
18. Blocks inspiratory gas flow, encourages maximum inspiration				
19. Repeats procedure for best patient effort				
20. Reassures patient; restores to prior status				
21. Calculates and interprets test results				
FOLLOW-UP				
22. Maintains/processes equipment				
23. Records pertinent data in chart and departmental records				
24. Notifies appropriate personnel				

STUDENT'S COMPREHENSION OF PROCEDURE (SELECT ONE ONLY)

The student demonstrates comprehensive knowledge of basic and advanced concepts beyond requirements of procedure	
The student demonstrates above average understanding of basic concepts applicable to the skill demonstrated	
The student demonstrates adequate knowledge of the essential elements of the task performed	
The student shows limited understanding of essential concepts related to the procedure	
The student has inadequate knowledge of even the basic concepts related to the task at hand	

OUTCOME CRITERIA (WHERE APPLICABLE)

	SPECIFY CRITERIA NOT MET AND/OR PERTINENT CONSTRAINTS
☐ MET	
☐ NOT MET	
☐ NOT APPL.	

ADDITIONAL COMMENTS

Include errors of omission or commission; if clinical therapeutic procedure emphasize communicative skills (verbal and non-verbal) and effectiveness of patient interaction:

SUMMARY PERFORMANCE EVALUATION AND RECOMMENDATIONS

SETTING	SATISFACTORY	UNSATISFACTORY	SPECIFY DEFICIENCIES
LABORATORY	☐ Can now perform skill under direct clinical supervision	☐ Requires additional laboratory practice	
CLINIC	☐ Ready for minimally supervised application and refinement	☐ Requires additional supervised clinical practice ☐ Complete re-evaluation required ☐ Re-evaluation·minor deficiencies only	

STUDENT: EVALUATOR: FACULTY:

STUDENT:	DATE:				

PROCEDURE (TASK): FORCED EXPIRATORY VOLUME

SETTING: ☐ LABORATORY ☐ OTHER: (SPECIFY) ☐ CLINIC		SATISFACTORY	UNSATISFACTORY	NOT OBSERVED	NOT APPLICABLE
CONDITIONS (DESCRIBE)					
EQUIPMENT UTILIZED:					

STEPS IN PROCEDURE OR TASK:

EQUIPMENT AND PATIENT PREPARATION				
1. Verifies, interprets, and evaluates physician's orders				
2. Selects, gathers, and assembles appropriate equipment				
3. Confirms the functional operation (calibrates) the measurement system				
4. Identifies patient, self, and department				
5. Obtains/assesses pertinent pulmonary history, physical findings, applicable laboratory data (enters appropriate data)				
6. Explains procedure and confirms patient understanding				
IMPLEMENTATION AND ASSESSMENT				
7. Connects patient to valve assembly (normal breathing)				
8. Initiates valve function				
9. Has patient take full inspiration/coordinates changeover				
10. Elicits forced/full expiration to residual volume (RV)				
11. Reassures patient				
12. Assesses test outcomes for reliability/validity				
13. Repeat procedure for best results/checks repeatibility				
14. Performs inspiratory capacity (IC), expiratory reserve volume (ERV)				
15. Performs maximum voluntary ventilation maneuver (MVV)				
16. Administers bronchodilator/waits for effect				
17. Repeats applicable procedures				
18. Calculates (obtains) patient, predicted, percent predicted values				
FOLLOW-UP				
19. Maintains/processes equipment				
20. Records pertinent data in chart and departmental records				
21. Notifies appropriate personnel				

STUDENT'S COMPREHENSION OF PROCEDURE (SELECT ONE ONLY)

The student demonstrates comprehensive knowledge of basic and advanced concepts beyond requirements of procedure	
The student demonstrates above average understanding of basic concepts applicable to the skill demonstrated	
The student demonstrates adequate knowledge of the essential elements of the task performed	
The student shows limited understanding of essential concepts related to the procedure	
The student has inadequate knowledge of even the basic concepts related to the task at hand	

OUTCOME CRITERIA (WHERE APPLICABLE)

☐ MET	SPECIFY CRITERIA NOT MET AND/OR PERTINENT CONSTRAINTS
☐ NOT MET	
☐ NOT APPL.	

ADDITIONAL COMMENTS

Include errors of omission or commission; if clinical therapeutic procedure emphasize communicative skills (verbal and non-verbal) and effectiveness of patient interaction:

SUMMARY PERFORMANCE EVALUATION AND RECOMMENDATIONS

SETTING	SATISFACTORY	UNSATISFACTORY	SPECIFY DEFICIENCIES
LABORATORY	☐ Can now perform skill under direct clinical supervision	☐ Requires additional laboratory practice	
CLINIC	☐ Ready for minimally supervised application and refinement	☐ Requires additional supervised clinical practice ☐ Complete re-evaluation required ☐ Re-evaluation·minor deficiencies only	

STUDENT: EVALUATOR: FACULTY:

STUDENT:	DATE:				

PROCEDURE (TASK): FUNCTIONAL RESIDUAL CAPACITY

	SATISFACTORY	UNSATISFACTORY	NOT OBSERVED	NOT APPLICABLE
SETTING: ☐ LABORATORY ☐ OTHER: (SPECIFY) ☐ CLINIC				
CONDITIONS (DESCRIBE)				
EQUIPMENT UTILIZED:				

STEPS IN PROCEDURE OR TASK:

EQUIPMENT AND PATIENT PREPARATION				
1. Verifies, interprets, and evaluates physician's orders				
2. Selects, gathers, and assembles appropriate equipment				
3. Confirms the functional operation (calibrates) the measurement system				
4. Identifies patient, self, and department				
5. Obtains/assesses pertinent pulmonary history, physical findings applicable laboratory data (enters appropriate data)				
6. Explains procedure and confirms patient understanding				
IMPLEMENTATION AND ASSESSMENT				
7. Adds gas mixture to bell/reservoir; reads value(s)				
8. Connects patient to valve assembly				
9. Open valve at functional residual capacity/provides oxygen flow				
10. Elicits normal breathing by patient				
11. Checks gas concentrations at determined intervals				
12. Reassures patient				
13. Proceeds with test until equilibration; reads value(s)				
14. Restores patient to normal breathing				
15. Assesses test outcome for reliability/validity				
16. Calculates (obtains) patient, predicted, percent predicted values for appropriate volumes/capacities				
FOLLOW-UP				
17. Maintains/processes equipment				
18. Records pertinent data in chart and department records				
19. Notifies appropriate personnel				

STUDENT'S COMPREHENSION OF PROCEDURE (SELECT ONE ONLY)

The student demonstrates comprehensive knowledge of basic and advanced concepts beyond requirements of procedure	
The student demonstrates above average understanding of basic concepts applicable to the skill demonstrated	
The student demonstrates adequate knowledge of the essential elements of the task performed	
The student shows limited understanding of essential concepts related to the procedure	
The student has inadequate knowledge of even the basic concepts related to the task at hand	

OUTCOME CRITERIA (WHERE APPLICABLE)

☐ MET	SPECIFY CRITERIA NOT MET AND/OR PERTINENT CONSTRAINTS
☐ NOT MET	
☐ NOT APPL.	

ADDITIONAL COMMENTS

Include errors of omission or commission; if clinical therapeutic procedure emphasize communicative skills (verbal and non-verbal) and effectiveness of patient interaction:

SUMMARY PERFORMANCE EVALUATION AND RECOMMENDATIONS

SETTING	SATISFACTORY	UNSATISFACTORY	SPECIFY DEFICIENCIES
LABORATORY	☐ Can now perform skill under direct clinical super-vision	☐ Requires additional laboratory practice	

CLINIC	☐ Ready for min-imally supervised application and refinement	☐ Requires additional supervised clinical practice
		  ☐ Complete re-evaluation required
		  ☐ Re-evaluation·minor deficiencies only	

STUDENT: EVALUATOR: FACULTY:

STUDENT:		DATE:				

PROCEDURE (TASK): DIFFUSING CAPACITY

	SATISFACTORY	UNSATISFACTORY	NOT OBSERVED	NOT APPLICABLE
SETTING: ☐ LABORATORY ☐ OTHER: (SPECIFY) ☐ CLINIC				
CONDITIONS (DESCRIBE)				
EQUIPMENT UTILIZED:				

STEPS IN PROCEDURE OR TASK:

	SATISFACTORY	UNSATISFACTORY	NOT OBSERVED	NOT APPLICABLE
EQUIPMENT AND PATIENT PREPARATION				
1. Verifies, interprets, and evaluates physician's order				
2. Selects, gathers, and assembles appropriate equipment				
3. Confirms the functional operation (calibrates) the measurement system				
4. Identifies patient, self, and department				
5. Obtains/assesses pertinent pulmonary history, physical findings, applicable laboratory data (enters appropriate data)				
6. Explains procedure and confirms patient understanding				
IMPLEMENTATION AND ASSESSMENT				
7. Fills carbon monoxide reservoir				
8. Connects patient to valve assembly				
9. Has patient exhale fully				
10. Initiates valve function				
11. Has patient take a full inspiration				
12. Ensures inspiratory hold for necessary time				
13. Collects sample during (slowed) patient exhalation				
14. Reads/records results; reassures patient				
15. Assesses test outcome for reliability/validity				
16. Repeat procedure if necessary				
17. Calculates test results				
FOLLOW-UP				
18. Maintains/processes equipment				
19. Records pertinent data in chart and department records				
20. Notifies appropriate personnel				

STUDENT'S COMPREHENSION OF PROCEDURE (SELECT ONE ONLY)

The student demonstrates comprehensive knowledge of basic and advanced concepts beyond requirements of procedure	
The student demonstrates above average understanding of basic concepts applicable to the skill demonstrated	
The student demonstrates adequate knowledge of the essential elements of the task performed	
The student shows limited understanding of essential concepts related to the procedure	
The student has inadequate knowledge of even the basic concepts related to the task at hand	

OUTCOME CRITERIA (WHERE APPLICABLE)

☐ MET	SPECIFY CRITERIA NOT MET AND/OR PERTINENT CONSTRAINTS
☐ NOT MET	
☐ NOT APPL.	

ADDITIONAL COMMENTS

Include errors of omission or commission; if clinical therapeutic procedure emphasize communicative skills (verbal and non-verbal) and effectiveness of patient interaction:

SUMMARY PERFORMANCE EVALUATION AND RECOMMENDATIONS

SETTING	SATISFACTORY	UNSATISFACTORY	SPECIFY DEFICIENCIES
LABORATORY	☐ Can now perform skill under direct clinical super-vision	☐ Requires additional laboratory practice	
CLINIC	☐ Ready for min-imally supervised application and refinement	☐ Requires additional supervised clinical practice ☐ Complete re-evaluation required ☐ Re-evaluation·minor deficiencies only	

STUDENT: EVALUATOR: FACULTY:

402

STUDENT:	DATE:				

PROCEDURE (TASK): ARTERIAL BLOOD GAS SAMPLING

SETTING: ☐ LABORATORY ☐ OTHER: (SPECIFY)
          ☐ CLINIC

CONDITIONS (DESCRIBE)

EQUIPMENT UTILIZED:

STEPS IN PROCEDURE OR TASK:	SATISFACTORY	UNSATISFACTORY	NOT OBSERVED	NOT APPLICABLE
EQUIPMENT AND PATIENT PREPARATION				
1. Washes hands				
2. Selects, gathers, and assembles appropriate equipment				
3. Verifies, interprets, and evaluates physician's order				
4. Checks chart for pertinent hematological information and compatibility of disease and procedure				
5. Identifies patient, self, and department				
6. Explains procedure and confirms patient understanding				
IMPLEMENTATION				
7. Tests for collateral circulation (Allen test)				
8. Prepares puncture site				
9. Prepares syringe (heparin)				
10. Palpates and anchors artery				
11. Reassures patient				
12. Penetrates artery, obtains sample				
13. Applies pressure to puncture site				
14. Caps syringe, ices sample				
15. Labels sample				
16. Reinspects puncture site				
17. Assures transportation and analysis of sample				
FOLLOW-UP				
18. Maintains/processes equipment				
19. Records pertinent data in chart and departmental records				
20. Notifies appropriate personnel				

STUDENT'S COMPREHENSION OF PROCEDURE (SELECT ONE ONLY)

The student demonstrates comprehensive knowledge of basic and advanced concepts beyond requirements of procedure	
The student demonstrates above average understanding of basic concepts applicable to the skill demonstrated	
The student demonstrates adequate knowledge of the essential elements of the task performed	
The student shows limited understanding of essential concepts related to the procedure	
The student has inadequate knowledge of even the basic concepts related to the task at hand	

OUTCOME CRITERIA (WHERE APPLICABLE)

☐ MET	SPECIFY CRITERIA NOT MET AND/OR PERTINENT CONSTRAINTS
☐ NOT MET	
☐ NOT APPL.	

ADDITIONAL COMMENTS

Include errors of omission or commission; if clinical therapeutic procedure emphasize communicative skills (verbal and non-verbal) and effectiveness of patient interaction:

SUMMARY PERFORMANCE EVALUATION AND RECOMMENDATIONS

SETTING	SATISFACTORY	UNSATISFACTORY	SPECIFY DEFICIENCIES
LABORATORY	☐ Can now perform skill under direct clinical super-vision	☐ Requires additional laboratory practice	
CLINIC	☐ Ready for min-imally supervised application and refinement	☐ Requires additional supervised clinical practice 　☐ Complete re-evaluation required 　☐ Re-evaluation·minor deficiencies only	

STUDENT:　　　　　EVALUATOR:　　　　FACULTY:

STUDENT:	DATE:

PROCEDURE (TASK): ARTERIAL BLOOD GAS ANALYSIS

SETTING: ☐ LABORATORY ☐ OTHER: (SPECIFY)
　　　　　 ☐ CLINIC

CONDITIONS (DESCRIBE)

EQUIPMENT UTILIZED:

STEPS IN PROCEDURE OR TASK:	SATISFACTORY	UNSATISFACTORY	NOT OBSERVED	NOT APPLICABLE
EQUIPMENT PREPARATION				
1. Activates analyzer, provides warm-up				
2. Inspects electrodes, analysis chamber				
3. Assures patency/function of fluid and gas lines				
4. Gathers necessary solutions and controls				
5. Calculates calibrating gas partial pressures (enters data)				
6. Balances/slopes pH and gas electrodes				
7. Confirms accuracy with control values				
IMPLEMENTATION				
8. Repeats balance calibration				
9. Mixes sample				
10. Introduces sample into analysis chamber				
11. Reads and records appropriate parameters				
12. Flushes analysis chamber				
FOLLOW-UP				
13. Calculates derived parameters				
14. Records results in departmental records				
15. Notifies appropriate personnel				
16. Maintains/processes equipment				

STUDENT'S COMPREHENSION OF PROCEDURE (SELECT ONE ONLY)

The student demonstrates comprehensive knowledge of basic and advanced concepts beyond requirements of procedure	
The student demonstrates above average understanding of basic concepts applicable to the skill demonstrated	
The student demonstrates adequate knowledge of the essential elements of the task performed ·	
The student shows limited understanding of essential concepts related to the procedure	
The student has inadequate knowledge of even the basic concepts related to the task at hand	

OUTCOME CRITERIA (WHERE APPLICABLE)

	SPECIFY CRITERIA NOT MET AND/OR PERTINENT CONSTRAINTS
☐ MET	
☐ NOT MET	
☐ NOT APPL.	

ADDITIONAL COMMENTS

Include errors of omission or commission; if clinical therapeutic procedure emphasize communicative skills (verbal and non-verbal) and effectiveness of patient interaction:

SUMMARY PERFORMANCE EVALUATION AND RECOMMENDATIONS

SETTING	SATISFACTORY	UNSATISFACTORY	SPECIFY DEFICIENCIES
LABORATORY	☐ Can now perform skill under direct clinical supervision	☐ Requires additional laboratory practice	
CLINIC	☐ Ready for minimally supervised application and refinement	☐ Requires additional supervised clinical practice ☐ Complete re-evaluation required ☐ Re-evaluation·minor deficiencies only	

STUDENT: EVALUATOR: FACULTY:

STUDENT:	DATE:

PROCEDURE (TASK): VENTILATOR PREPARATION AND APPLICATION

	SATISFACTORY	UNSATISFACTORY	NOT OBSERVED	NOT APPLICABLE
SETTING: ☐ LABORATORY ☐ OTHER: (SPECIFY) ☐ CLINIC				
CONDITIONS (DESCRIBE)				
EQUIPMENT UTILIZED:				

STEPS IN PROCEDURE OR TASK:

	SATISFACTORY	UNSATISFACTORY	NOT OBSERVED	NOT APPLICABLE
EQUIPMENT PREPARATION				
1. Washes hands				
2. Verifies, interprets, and evaluates physician's orders				
3. Selects, gathers, and assembles ventilator and circuitry				
4. Fills humidifier with sterile, distilled water				
5. Completes operational check of ventilator function				
6. Determines appropriate mode of ventilation				
7. Determines and sets appropriate ventilatory parameters				
8. Sets initial flowrate for proper inspiratory/expiratory rate				
PATIENT PREPARATION				
9. Identifies patient, self, and department				
10. Explains procedure and confirms patient understanding				
IMPLEMENTATION AND ASSESSMENT				
11. Attaches patient to ventilator during expiration				
12. Sets all alarm functions				
13. Confirms ventilator rate (patient spontaneous rate)				
14. Assesses patient response				
15. Draws or has drawn an arterial blood gas				
16. Readjusts parameters according to blood gas data				
17. Repeats steps 13 - 15 until patient stabilized				
FOLLOW-UP				
18. Maintains/processes equipment				
19. Records pertinent data in chart and departmental records				
20. Notifies appropriate personnel				

STUDENT'S COMPREHENSION OF PROCEDURE (SELECT ONE ONLY)

The student demonstrates comprehensive knowledge of basic and advanced concepts beyond requirements of procedure	
The student demonstrates above average understanding of basic concepts applicable to the skill demonstrated	
The student demonstrates adequate knowledge of the essential elements of the task performed	
The student shows limited understanding of essential concepts related to the procedure	
The student has inadequate knowledge of even the basic concepts related to the task at hand	

OUTCOME CRITERIA (WHERE APPLICABLE)

☐ MET	SPECIFY CRITERIA NOT MET AND/OR PERTINENT CONSTRAINTS
☐ NOT MET	
☐ NOT APPL.	

ADDITIONAL COMMENTS

Include errors of omission or commission; if clinical therapeutic procedure emphasize communicative skills (verbal and non-verbal) and effectiveness of patient interaction:

SUMMARY PERFORMANCE EVALUATION AND RECOMMENDATIONS

SETTING	SATISFACTORY	UNSATISFACTORY	SPECIFY DEFICIENCIES
LABORATORY	☐ Can now perform skill under direct clinical supervision	☐ Requires additional laboratory practice	
CLINIC	☐ Ready for minimally supervised application and refinement	☐ Requires additional supervised clinical practice ☐ Complete re-evaluation required ☐ Re-evaluation·minor deficiencies only	

STUDENT: EVALUATOR: FACULTY:

STUDENT:	DATE:				

PROCEDURE (TASK): ROUTINE VENTILATOR CHECK

SETTING: ☐ LABORATORY ☐ OTHER: (SPECIFY) ☐ CLINIC	SATISFACTORY	UNSATISFACTORY	NOT OBSERVED	NOT APPLICABLE
CONDITIONS (DESCRIBE)				
EQUIPMENT UTILIZED:				

STEPS IN PROCEDURE OR TASK:

EQUIPMENT AND PATIENT PREPARATION				
1. Washes hands				
2. Selects, gathers, and assembles appropriate equipment				
3. Verifies, interprets, and evaluates physician's order				
4. Identifies patient, self, and department				
5. Explains procedure and confirms patient understanding				
IMPLEMENTATION AND ASSESSMENT				
6. Verifies current ventilator settings				
7. Checks humidifier function and water level				
8. Refills humidifier				
9. Checks airway temperature				
10. Checks circuit integrity for leaks/obstructions and position				
11. Inspects and assesses patient status				
12. Correlates pre-set values with those monitored				
13. Ensures proper ventilator function (troubleshoots)				
14. Verifies all alarms functions/settings				
15. Reassures patient				
FOLLOW-UP				
16. Maintains/processes equipment				
17. Records pertinent data in chart and departmental records				
18. Notifies appropriate personnel				

STUDENT'S COMPREHENSION OF PROCEDURE (SELECT ONE ONLY)

The student demonstrates comprehensive knowledge of basic and advanced concepts beyond requirements of procedure	
The student demonstrates above average understanding of basic concepts applicable to the skill demonstrated	
The student demonstrates adequate knowledge of the essential elements of the task performed	
The student shows limited understanding of essential concepts related to the procedure	
The student has inadequate knowledge of even the basic concepts related to the task at hand	

OUTCOME CRITERIA (WHERE APPLICABLE)

☐ MET	SPECIFY CRITERIA NOT MET AND/OR PERTINENT CONSTRAINTS
☐ NOT MET	
☐ NOT APPL.	

ADDITIONAL COMMENTS

Include errors of omission or commission; if clinical therapeutic procedure emphasize communicative skills (verbal and non-verbal) and effectiveness of patient interaction:

SUMMARY PERFORMANCE EVALUATION AND RECOMMENDATIONS

SETTING	SATISFACTORY	UNSATISFACTORY	SPECIFY DEFICIENCIES
LABORATORY	☐ Can now perform skill under direct clinical super-vision	☐ Requires additional laboratory practice	

CLINIC	☐ Ready for min-imally supervised application and refinement	☐ Requires additional supervised clinical practice
		  ☐ Complete re-evaluation required
		  ☐ Re-evaluation·minor deficiencies only	

STUDENT: EVALUATOR: FACULTY:

STUDENT:	DATE:				

PROCEDURE (TASK): IMV, WEANING, VENTILATOR DISCONTINUANCE

SETTING: ☐ LABORATORY ☐ OTHER: (SPECIFY) ☐ CLINIC	SATISFACTORY	UNSATISFACTORY	NOT OBSERVED	NOT APPLICABLE
CONDITIONS (DESCRIBE)				
EQUIPMENT UTILIZED:				

STEPS IN PROCEDURE OR TASK:

EQUIPMENT AND PATIENT PREPARATION				
1. Washes hands				
2. Selects, gathers, and assembles appropriate equipment				
3. Verifies, interprets, and evaluates physician's order				
4. Identifies patient, self, and department				
5. Explains procedure and confirms patient understanding				
IMPLEMENTATION AND ASSESSMENT				
6. Obtains baseline physiological profile				
7. Performs operational check of equipment function				
8. Reassures patient				
9. Initiates IMV mode (weaning procedure)				
10. Assesses patient's response				
11. Readjusts therapy as indicated (reassures patient)				
12. Monitors patient progress				
FOLLOW-UP				
13. Provides appropriate follow-up care				
14. Records pertinent data in chart and departmental records				
15. Maintains/processes equipment				
16. Notifies appropriate personnel				

411

STUDENT'S COMPREHENSION OF PROCEDURE (SELECT ONE ONLY)

The student demonstrates comprehensive knowledge of basic and advanced concepts beyond requirements of procedure	
The student demonstrates above average understanding of basic concepts applicable to the skill demonstrated	
The student demonstrates adequate knowledge of the essential elements of the task performed	
The student shows limited understanding of essential concepts related to the procedure	
The student has inadequate knowledge of even the basic concepts related to the task at hand	

OUTCOME CRITERIA (WHERE APPLICABLE)

☐ MET	SPECIFY CRITERIA NOT MET AND/OR PERTINENT CONSTRAINTS
☐ NOT MET	
☐ NOT APPL.	

ADDITIONAL COMMENTS

Include errors of omission or commission; if clinical therapeutic procedure emphasize communicative skills (verbal and non-verbal) and effectiveness of patient interaction:

SUMMARY PERFORMANCE EVALUATION AND RECOMMENDATIONS

SETTING	SATISFACTORY	UNSATISFACTORY	SPECIFY DEFICIENCIES
LABORATORY	☐ Can now perform skill under direct clinical super-vision	☐ Requires additional laboratory practice	

CLINIC	☐ Ready for min-imally supervised application and refinement	☐ Requires additional supervised clinical practice
		   ☐ Complete re-evaluation required
		   ☐ Re-evaluation·minor deficiencies only	

STUDENT: EVALUATOR: FACULTY:

STUDENT:	DATE:

PROCEDURE (TASK): CONTINUOUS DISTENDING PRESSURE THERAPY

SETTING: ☐ LABORATORY ☐ OTHER: (SPECIFY)
        ☐ CLINIC

CONDITIONS (DESCRIBE)

EQUIPMENT UTILIZED:

STEPS IN PROCEDURE OR TASK:	SATISFACTORY	UNSATISFACTORY	NOT OBSERVED	NOT APPLICABLE
EQUIPMENT AND PATIENT PREPARATION				
1. Washes hands				
2. Selects, gathers, and assembles appropriate equipment				
3. Verifies, interprets, and evaluates physician's order				
4. Identifies patient, self, and department				
5. Explains procedure and confirms patient's understanding				
IMPLEMENTATION AND ASSESSMENT				
6. Obtains baseline physiological profile				
7. Performs operational check of equipment function				
8. Reassures patient				
9. Initiates continuous distending pressure				
10. Ensures appropriate pressure level				
11. Assesses patient's response				
12. Readjusts pressure to optimal level (reassures patient)				
13. Monitors patient progress				
FOLLOW-UP				
14. Provides appropriate follow-up care/monitoring				
15. Records pertinent data in chart and departmental records				
16. Maintains/processes equipment				
17. Notifies appropriate personnel				

STUDENT'S COMPREHENSION OF PROCEDURE (SELECT ONE ONLY)

The student demonstrates comprehensive knowledge of basic and advanced concepts beyond requirements of procedure	
The student demonstrates above average understanding of basic concepts applicable to the skill demonstrated	
The student demonstrates adequate knowledge of the essential elements of the task performed	
The student shows limited understanding of essential concepts related to the procedure	
The student has inadequate knowledge of even the basic concepts related to the task at hand	

OUTCOME CRITERIA (WHERE APPLICABLE)

☐ MET	SPECIFY CRITERIA NOT MET AND/OR PERTINENT CONSTRAINTS
☐ NOT MET	
☐ NOT APPL.	

ADDITIONAL COMMENTS

Include errors of omission or commission; if clinical therapeutic procedure emphasize communicative skills (verbal and non-verbal) and effectiveness of patient interaction:

SUMMARY PERFORMANCE EVALUATION AND RECOMMENDATIONS

SETTING	SATISFACTORY	UNSATISFACTORY	SPECIFY DEFICIENCIES
LABORATORY	☐ Can now perform skill under direct clinical supervision	☐ Requires additional laboratory practice	
CLINIC	☐ Ready for minimally supervised application and refinement	☐ Requires additional supervised clinical practice ☐ Complete re-evaluation required ☐ Re-evaluation·minor deficiencies only	

STUDENT: EVALUATOR: FACULTY: